COURAGE THROUGH CHRONIC DISEASE

COURAGE THROUGH CHRONIC DISEASE

Discovery, Hope, Transformation

Carolyn Humphreys, OCDS, OTR/L

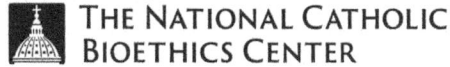
THE NATIONAL CATHOLIC BIOETHICS CENTER

Broomall, Pennsylvania

Published by
The National Catholic Bioethics Center
600 Reed Rd., Suite 102, Broomall, PA 19008
Printed in the United States

© The National Catholic Bioethics Center 2023

Permission has been granted for the partial reprinting of several articles published previously: Tony Snow, "Cancer's Unexpected Blessings," *Chritianity Today*, July 20, 2007, reprinted in "Tony Snow's Testimony," *Poetic Expressions* (blog), accessed September 20, 2022, https://www.poeticexpressions.co.uk/t-snow/, 67–59; Timothy Radcliffe, "A Spirituality of Suffering and Healing," *Religious Life Review* (September–October 2012), 159–160; Corrie ten Boom with Jamie Buckingham, *Tramp for the Lord* (Fort Washington, PA: CLC Publications, 1974), 55–57; Helen Steiner Rice, "There Are Blessings in Everything," in *The Poems and Prayers of Helen Steiner Rice*, (Fleming H. Revell, Baker Book House Company, 2003), 193–194.

No part of this publication may be reproduced, stored in a retrieval system, or transmitted, in any form or by any means, without the prior permission in writing of The National Catholic Bioethics Center, or as expressly permitted by law, by license, or under terms agreed upon with the appropriate reproduction rights organization. Inquiries concerning reproduction outside the scope of the above should be sent to The National Catholic Bioethics Center at the address above.

You must not circulate this work in any other form, and you must impose this same condition on any acquirer.

Library of Congress Control Number: 202394071

ISBN: 978-0-935372-78-6

Cover design by Nicholas Furton

Contents

Foreword..vii
Acknowledgements..ix
A Wake-up Call...1
Who Am I Now?...19
Aspects of Care..37
From Survivors to Pioneers.....................................53
The Elders among Us..67
The Emperor and the Children...............................81
Grief Revealed...97
Adjustments on the Road......................................111
Perseverance as the Motivator...............................127
The Essential Need for Respect.............................141
Finding Harmony..159
The Spiritual Dimension.......................................173

Foreword

The term chronic disease covers a wide realm of human dysfunction. The diagnoses include diabetes, heart conditions, traumatic brain injury, stroke, chronic pain, and various forms of arthritis, to name a few.

Courage through Chronic Disease: Discovery, Hope, Transformation takes the reader on a soul-searching journey. This moving experience explores all roads, avenues, streets, and boulevards of living with any type of chronic disease through a practical yet philosophical point of view. Each chapter reveals different aspects of the struggle an individual with a chronic condition may encounter through life's journey, and also gives practical suggestions for coping with the difficulties. The author offers thoughtful advice within the venues of religion, literature, and the experiences of real-life people.

The beginning of the book sets the stage for the journey with the initial awareness of a chronic disease through medical examination. From here, the reader is taken by the hand and lead to introspection on the meaning of personal identity.

One realizes that the person who lived yesterday may be very different from the one who lives today. Ideas are offered to explore, in a positive manner, this new identity, which include a balance between taking care of oneself and accepting help from others. There are answers to a multitude of questions. How can one become a better person while living with a chronic condition? What qualities should a caregiver have to be of the most benefit to a person with a chronic illness? How does one achieve a sense of well-being so as to develop the strength to move forward? How does one overcome specific obstacles when dealing with either childhood or adult cancers? How does one resolve an overwhelming sense of grief which may be caused by a chronic condition? How does one acknowledge the darkness and yet emerge through the light of life?

The book acknowledges the negative, but dwells on the positive. This is a book that allows the reader to move through the various stages of accepting a chronic disease. The ultimate goal is that the reader discovers unknown strengths to build a wellspring of positive hope, in order to create a transformation into a life filled with quality and satisfaction, and create a harmonic sense of spiritual and sustainable faith.

Tina Scott Shadley, OTR/L
Home Health Occupational Therapist

Acknowledgements

This book would not have come to fruition without helpful suggestions and good advice from several people. I am very grateful for, and highly appreciative of, those who helped make this book possible: Peggy Normandin, Sr. Anna O'Reilly, DMJ, Sassan Farjami, MD, Barbara Harrend, OCDS, RN, Pauline Chapman, Judy Cooper, OCDS, Ida Rubin, OCDS, and Fr. James Kubicki, SJ. They excel in their fields of interest and added quality and wisdom to the text. A special thank you is given to Tina Scott Shadley, OTR/L, who has had years of experience in home health. Her foreword and text review were invaluable.

Chapter 1

A Wake-up Call

Michael Richard "Rich" Clifford was born on October 13, 1952, in California and raised in Utah. In high school, he excelled in chemistry and wanted to be a chemist. But in July 1969, his ambitions abruptly changed when Neil Armstrong walked on the moon. Rich wanted to be an astronaut too. In June 1974, Rich graduated from West Point with a bachelor's of science. As a second lieutenant, he served at Fort Carson, Colorado. He was the top graduate in his flight class at the Army aviation school and became an army aviator. For three years, he served as a service platoon commander in Nuremberg, West Germany. In 1982 he completed master's of science in aerospace engineering from the Georgia Institute of Technology and became an assistant professor of mechanical engineering at West Point.

He graduated from Naval Test Pilot School in 1986 and became an experimental test pilot and master army aviator, but his end goal was still to be an astronaut. He was selected for NASA's Space Shuttle program in 1990 and two years later flew his first shuttle mission. In 1994, after his second shuttle mission, Rich underwent a routine physical examination, which revealed the beginning stages of Parkinson's disease, an incurable neurodegenerative condition marked by trembling limbs, rigid muscles, and a shuffling gait. After months of tests, the physicians cleared him to fly. Since the doctors said he could still do his job competently, he told only his wife, sons, shuttle commander, and limited NASA crew about the diagnosis. From May 1994 to September 1995, he worked as the lead for space station vehicle and assembly issues. He was a veteran of three space flights and logged 665 hours in space, including a six-hour flawless space walk. In 1995, with the rank of lieutenant colonel, he retired from the Army. Rich left NASA in 1997 and worked for Boeing as director of operations and training for the International Space Station and then as deputy program manager for the Space Shuttle program. He is now retired, and even though his symptoms have progressed, he enjoys meeting other people with Parkinson's, sharing his story, and encouraging them not give up on life.

Rich Clifford led a very active life and did not imagine he would contract Parkinson's disease. He shows us that life is a mystery. We think we have all the time in the world. We have long-range plans, places to go, and things to do. We have no significant problems. Our job is rewarding, our family is pleasant, our home is comfortable, and we are proud of our accomplishments and our physical health. All is going well according to our standards, but will this remain so? We know life's circumstances can change in an instant or, as in Rich's case, over time.

A Wake-up Call

What Is Chronic Disease?

A physical chronic disease is a health condition that persists and requires ongoing attention. Chronic diseases have increased because of advances in health care, longer life spans, and a change from fatal to manageable diseases. A chronic disease is usually prolonged or lifelong and may have no known cause or cure. Nevertheless, many chronic diseases are treatable. Although the terms disease and illness are used interchangeably, they are different. Diseases are usually lifelong and require management, while illnesses are usually short-term and can be cured. A disease is not as easy to deal with or to care for as is an illness. An acute illness usually has a distinct beginning, middle, and end with a return to the same level of health as before the onset of the illness. Because of complications, symptoms that come and go, long-term prognosis, and progression of the disease, chronic diseases do not seem to have the clarity or distinct treatments of acute illnesses. A disease can remain the same, be in remission, steadily get worse, or be cyclical.

The most common chronic condition, of which people may not be aware, is hypertension. Other common diseases include rheumatoid arthritis, chronic fatigue syndrome, Crohn's disease, fibromyalgia, and atherosclerosis. If we develop a chronic disease before the age of twenty, it can be called juvenile, as in juvenile diabetes or juvenile rheumatoid arthritis. Although they are unwanted, most of us will develop one or more chronic diseases during our adult life. However, not all of them entail physical pain. Even though chronic diseases cannot be cured, they need not be a dominant factor in our lives if they are managed appropriately.

Responding to the Challenge

The onset of a physical chronic disease is a common change. It can happen as suddenly as overnight or gradually develop over the years. Whatever the onset, we are not the person we used to be. Things are not quite the same. We must pay attention to our chronic disease needs because, if we do not, they will eventually take their toll. Since a chronic condition requires dependence on doctors and others, we are no longer ruggedly independent. Moreover, life becomes fragile and frightening when we cannot name the disease that is prompting the symptoms we are experiencing or when we do not know anything about the disease after it is diagnosed. When we do not know what is wrong, we are afraid. Our feelings can be raw and easily stirred up, and our imagination can run wild with worst-case scenarios.

To avoid imagining things, especially the worst and the morbid, the first priority is to get a definitive diagnosis. Before visiting the doctor, it is important to write down all apparent symptoms, how often they occur, how long they last, and uncommon incidents that do not appear to be disease related. A list is valuable because, while waiting for the doctor, we may think some symptoms have disappeared or some things are not worth talking about. An accurate diagnosis may take a long time because it can involve interviews, observations, blood tests and other assays, scans, and whatever else is needed. We may be asked to see different doctors or go to a university medical center. These are unexpected, unwelcome interruptions in our familiar daily routine. Diagnostic activities can be times of high stress, and we can burst into tears because of fear, anxiety, or confusion or for no apparent reason.

A Wake-up Call

When we receive an accurate diagnosis, it can alleviate built-up stress. There is some relief. The unknown is now known. Our symptoms have a cause. Yet we wonder about new concerns. We ruminate about the possible effects of our chronic disease. Will it diminish us, make us a second-class citizen, an outsider, or a broken or useless person? We can really bombard ourselves with self-defeating images.

However, time will reveal that having a chronic disease does not mean we will become any of these things. Negative ruminations are a natural reaction, but they make coping more difficult. These thoughts occur more frequently during the early years but diminish in time as care for the disease becomes daily routine. A good practice is to strive to remain liberated from pessimistic thoughts and downbeat people, focus on the best in ourselves, and develop our creative gifts that sustain goodness and love.

In the beginning, our chronic disease may be our primary focus, but as time goes on, we move beyond that perspective. Our life has not ended; it just takes a new direction as habits and routines are adjusted to address our current needs. In time our disease takes its proper place and becomes incorporated into our routine. We learn to live more courageously and deal with things, like walking, which the average person takes for granted. We are not a diseased person; we are a person who happens to have a disease. And it is well known that diminishment in some areas can open the way to discoveries in other areas. Who we become is more vital than who we were.

When health concerns settle into their appropriate place in our lifestyle, we are defined not by what happens to us, but by who we are as unique, valuable individuals. We can become better than we were before our diagnosis. A chronic disorder can teach us to "take the bull by the horns" throughout life. This phrase is based on the idea that holding a bull by his horns is a courageous and direct action that means we deal bravely and decisively with anything that is difficult, dangerous, or unpleasant. In chronic conditions, we deal with a specific matter in a direct manner; we confront a difficulty rather than deny or avoid it: "We choose to go to the moon in this decade and do the other things, not because they are easy, but because they are hard."[1] In spite of frustrations and fear, we can navigate our journey with chronic disease and find that life is worth living. Helen Keller wrote, "Life is either a daring adventure or nothing. ... Character cannot be developed in ease and quiet. Only through experience of trial and suffering can the soul be strengthened, ambition inspired, and success achieved."[2]

A Time to Pause

We live *in hac lacrimarum valle*, in this valley of tears. Chronic disease can result in not being able to do something we were able to do before and, if it is degenerative, can include more losses as the years pass. There can be a change from being invincibly independent to being minimally or severely dependent. If we were fiercely independent before onset, it will be difficult to accept needing assistance in whatever form it takes. Assistance means a certain reliance on others for our physical needs and therefore decreased self-sufficiency. Yet if we think about it, is anyone really independent? Who doesn't need an electrician, plumber, computer technician, or

A Wake-up Call

auto mechanic? Our lives are dependent on others and subject to circumstances beyond our control.

No two people experience life, or their chronic disease, in the same way. A chronic disease diagnosis can cause us to stop and reevaluate what is most important in our day and what means most to us. We can no longer kid ourselves. We may not feel, think, or act like we used to. There may be role reversals and lost dreams. However, as we let go of our former self-perceptions, we can forge a new sense of who we are and what we can do. It is time to reorient and renew ourselves. We gracefully move from a focus on our disease to a focus on living. We can change the way we think about ourselves. Although we may not have a choice regarding our loss, we can choose to pull through it: "All we have to do is look around us and we see that loss is one half of the process of life. New life can only come when there is a letting go of what was there before. This is the story of human existence from beginning to end."[3]

Some chronic diseases are not visible to others. A person with a no-show disease appears to be in good health. Non-visible diseases include fibromyalgia, high blood pressure, high cholesterol, early stage heart disease, diabetes, and uterine cancer. Conversely, a chronic disease may be obvious through a physical deformity; the use of a cane, wheelchair, brace, or splint; or anything we can see. Certain long-term physical conditions can progress to needing personal assistance in daily activities such as hygiene, dressing, grooming, and eating. A chronic disease can result in at least one limitation in activities of daily living. Physical limitations can range from needing help with a fine motor task, like threading a needle because of a hand tremor, to being bedbound from a stroke. A long-term disease can affect one body system or be systemic, affecting several body systems. A chronic physical disease requires periodic visits to the doctor and can have daily responsibilities such as medications or times for rest. It can reduce our level of activity, change our physical abilities, require diet restrictions, cause fatigue or muscle weakness, decrease range of motion, or limit mobility. Full-time employment may be reduced to part-time, or a home may need modifications. However, as we learn to deal with big and small issues, we can become stronger for it.

People with disabilities should not be defined primarily by what they cannot do. The limitation or disease is a peripheral element. What is central is a person's unique identity. We learn to cope with our disease, and down the road, coping becomes second nature. Someone may be disabled and have a magnetic personality, a well-honed talent, or a beautiful smile. A person does not need a totally functioning body to enjoy life or be loveable. An individual with a physical disability can be a well-integrated person and a blessing to society. We can see this in Rich Clifford and his Parkinson's disease.

Embrace the Lighter Side

An elderly gentleman named George had a stroke and went to a center for rehabilitation. After discharge, his occupational therapist went to his home to do an initial assessment. This was in the middle of July, and it was extremely hot outside. George met his occupational therapist at the door in a thick sweat suit, perspiring heavily. Come to find out, when he was admitted to the rehab center, he was told that he had to wear sweat suits. This was for ease of dressing while he exercised at the center. He thought he had to wear sweat suits for the rest of his life because he had a stroke. He was one happy person when his occupational therapist suggested he change into shorts and a T-shirt. Because he no longer needed to wear a sweat suit, he grinned like a Cheshire cat all day.

In Proverbs 17:22, King Solomon says, "A cheerful heart is a good medicine, but a downcast spirit dries up the bones." Dealing with a chronic disease can indeed give us periods of dry bones, but with the gift of humor, we can reinvigorate them. Finding humor in difficult situations is a lifesaver. Laughter preserves our sanity when dealing with difficult situations. It safeguards our dignity during undignified situations when we receive help from others or do things that are tedious and time consuming. Telling a funny joke can divert our thoughts from pain, keep our heart young, poke good fun at the embarrassments of a disease, or bring a smile to a disappointing situation. A playful or mischievous sense of humor can release pent-up frustration or break the ice for those who are ill at ease when they are with seriously sick people. Laughter is priceless. It alleviates daily annoyances that come with a chronic disease. It has a way of neutralizing the influence of one's disease by giving the person more command, by decreasing unwanted sympathy, and by offering a constructive alternative to chronic complaints. Mirth decreases the effect of a chronic disease from its daily annoyances to its life altering events. Humor can help us look at a negative situation in a new way or understand it from a different viewpoint. By seeing new lights, we refrain from being trapped in the dark of troubling situations.

Positive humor is simple and fun loving. Who can forget those ubiquitous knock-knock jokes? "Knock knock" "Who's there?" "A broken pencil." "A broken pencil who?" "Never mind, it's pointless." Cartoons, comics, or TV shows can also be the pause that refreshes. A good rule is to find something that is humorous each day. If we are receptive to the lighter moments, it will balance life's ironies and incongruences. We are all a little bit goofy and need to laugh at our silliness, especially when things get too serious.

Practical Steps for Coping with Chronic Disease

Practical help makes life easier. We must respect our own limitations and pain thresholds. In other words, stop or revise a task before you get exhausted or if it provokes pain that lasts for more than twenty minutes after the task is completed. Conversely, avoid taking advantage of people. Do not rely on overly helpful relatives or friends to do things that you can do yourself. Find alternative ways of doing things that are difficult because of your disease. You show respect for yourself when you work within the new boundaries of what you can accomplish. Household tasks can be redistributed to preserve your energy: Are there any that can be done less frequently or in an easier or more efficient way? Is a high-energy activity followed by a low-energy one? Do you rush through a task just to get to the next one, or do you complete it at your own pace and celebrate its completion? Our abilities and resources need to balance our expectations and desires. We find the mean between going too fast and going too slow, doing too much and doing too little, resting and exercising, working and playing, and praying and planning.

Stay up-to-date about managing your disease because treatments may improve and our needs at onset may change or be different several years later. Never has so much information about diseases and their related matters been available to us. However, cautiously screen information and ads that promise fast relief or the latest remedy or cure. To maintain a gentle acceptance of your chronic disease is to embrace wherever you are on the disease continuum. In other words, accept things as they are rather than as you would like them to be. As you look back on your years with a chronic disease, somehow you can sense that pain can be a channel for growth in ways you were unaware.

A chronic disease can cultivate a tough yet compassionate resolve, and over time we will develop an increased tolerance toward people who say odd things to us. For instance, a woman who uses a walker is at a restaurant with her friend. A young waiter asks her friend what the woman would like to eat, assuming wrongly that, because she uses a walker, she is not capable of ordering for herself. The woman thinks, "Everyone has limitations." Most likely, the waiter has not had any significant contact with someone who uses a walker and saw the walker and not the woman. It is up to her to kindly teach him—people use walkers to walk just like they use forks to eat. Similarly, when people respond glibly to an assistive device by saying something like "keep smiling," perhaps it is because they really do not know what to say and feel they should say something. They hope their words, although seemingly superficial, will help in some way. In reality they may feel as helpless as we do concerning the things that cannot be changed, and they may care for us beyond the expression of words. There was a time when many people had long-term relationships with their family doctor. He knew them and their families well. Today, however, with the limited amount of time physicians spend with us, and care being distributed among several specialists, we need to actively participate in our health care. Being an active partner is more beneficial than being a passive patient. We are proactive by maintaining a dynamic attitude in managing and understanding our disease.

A team approach works well in health care. It can give the patient an active voice when communicating with health care professionals. The members of our team are our health care partners. Doctors are our primary partners. We follow their advice and ask questions as needed. Other members of our team can be a physical therapist, occupational therapist, psychologist, social worker, nurse practitioner, or caregiver. They too are contacted as needed. Within our health care team, we are the captain, as well as the case manager, regarding the care we desire. However, we neither overstate nor understate our own importance. We are team players. If we look at our team as human beings first, it is easier to see ourselves as a working partner with the others.

We need to pull our own weight regarding our health care and not depend on our doctors to fix everything, or to make our decisions, while we do nothing. The time a doctor spends with us is limited, so we use it wisely by organizing our thoughts, asking questions, and writing down answers. We raise concerns at the beginning of a visit instead of at the end. It is important that we like, trust, and respect our doctors. If we do not feel a sound connection to our doctor, we need to find another one. If we have several doctors, we keep them updated about the current status of our condition and changes in medication. We maintain responsibility by keeping our medical appointments and learning about the medications we have been prescribed. We need to be responsible because the final decisions about our health care are up to us.

The Spiritual Realm

We must realize medicine's limitations. There is not a cure for everything. Some things cannot be fixed. More treatment is not always better. Sometimes there are no answers, and the best that can be done is to control the symptoms. However, healing is more than cure or symptom relief. It includes the ability to find new strengths, to learn more about ourselves, and to abide by sound guidance regarding well-being and the sacred quality of life. Even though we have frail physical health, we can excel in mental and spiritual health. Everyone has spiritual needs, and it takes a courageous person to admit to them. A chronic condition can be a wake-up call, or a renewal call, to fully embrace the reality that God truly exists and that we travel in a spiritual as well as an earthly landscape. The beliefs and practices of faith grounded in a time-honored religion can shape and direct our lives. Deep roots are rarely set within a free-form spirituality that has ambiguous moral and social values and contains a diverse mix of beliefs and new age thinking. Incorporating the practices of religion into our lifestyle fosters and strengthens a sense of well-being, optimism, tranquility, and altruism. It increases our network of friends and encourages us to abide by authority, such as by following doctor's orders. A person who is serious about his or her religion is less likely to do harmful things such as smoke, drink to excess, or engage in promiscuous or violent behavior. It is well-known that people who regularly worship God lead longer and happier lives. Living without God, who is infinite and ineffable, is a severe impoverishment: "Everyone needs to be touched by the comfort and attraction of God's saving love, which is mysteriously at work in each person, above and beyond their faults and failings."[4]

The Bible tells us we are made in the image and likeness of God. Grace assists us in striving to maintain that image by reaching upward and outward toward what is beautiful, good, and true. A chronic condition may provide the time to reflect upon and practice this art of reaching up to God and out to others, especially in little ways, which are the best ways. In a spiritual context, living with a chronic disease reveals that life is more about sharing and helping than about getting and spending.

The most characteristic expression of authentic religions is prayer. In the Christian tradition, prayer invigorates as it helps to form a secure identity based on the life and love of Jesus, who shows us the way to God the Father and teaches us how to pray. Prayer helps us see things in a way that sustains life. Prayer can recharge low energy, be a balm for our wounds, or be a boost for work that needs to be done. Deep prayer can be a wordless union with God. With him in our lives, everything has a higher purpose, even if we do not find out what it is. No matter what our circumstances, we believe God's love surrounds us, enfolds us, and guides us toward our highest good. Prayer sustains our confidence in God and in ourselves.

Disease has been with us since the fall of humanity. By embracing the gift of faith, we can unite our suffering with Jesus's crucifixion and offer it to God the Father for the betterment of humanity. Faith in Jesus reveals that suffering is not useless. Rather, it brings new meaning to life. We see beyond a broken world. Jesus's teachings open our eyes to new ways of looking at things. We evolve from being indifferent about unfavorable aspects of life to thinking about how we can make them better. Learning about matters of faith is above and beyond reason. We may be drawn to investigate faith through academic pursuits, but faith in God continues to develop beyond the intellect. Many things on the spiritual journey cannot be fully explained or understood. Faith inspires us to live rightly and do good for others. It takes us into the deepest meaning of life and builds a strong relationship with God.

Faith gives us the assurance to never give up on hope. Like a bird that sings in the dark, a lighthouse in a storm, or a brilliant star in the night, hope is the beacon that guides us forward. Hope magnifies our vision to see brightness beyond the shadows and light beyond the dark. Like a sturdy vine that makes its way around obstacles and difficulties, hope is a strong companion on our journey. Faith and hope are like sturdy supports that keep us standing straight and moving forward.

Having a chronic disease does not decrease our value as human beings. More precisely, we can be remarkably resilient concerning our self-worth when we have a will to survive in the face of disease and when we perceive a horizon much larger than we see. At onset we can fume and fuss about our diagnosis, but in time we can gracefully accept and settle down to its reality. When something is taken away from us, perhaps it is making way for something better. We become peaceful about our diagnosis and limitations and strive to maintain an ongoing positive attitude toward our disease and ourselves. A chronic disease can be the push we need to develop healthier habits, to build inner strength, to learn new skills, or to search for a more profound meaning in life. How we handle the difficulties caused by our disease can be a source of inspiration to others. Because of our lifelong disease, we can do much good, since we know what it is like to need help. We can reach beyond our personal circumstances to a cause or mission greater than ourselves. Coping with a lifelong disease can give us insights into other people's pain, strengthen our empathy, and motivate us to help others. Each of us has special gifts to discover and use well: "I am only one; but still I am one. I cannot do everything; but still I can do something; and because I cannot do everything, I will not refuse to do the something I can do."[5]

This book does not offer diagnosis or treatment for specific chronic diseases, nor is it a source for medical advice, which is for doctors. The text goes beyond the medical model and addresses the different aspects of a well-integrated human being who is striving toward a dignified, respectful way of life and who happens to have a chronic disease. These pages invite readers to observe and improve their quality of life and strengthen the various components that make up their personhood. In spite of, or even because of, a chronic physical condition, we can move forward and become better people. Having confidence in God and in ourselves, and responding positively to grace, endorses us as valuable and distinctive human beings who are summoned to the fulfillment of incredible potential for greatness and achievement.

Notes

1. John F. Kennedy, "Moon Speech," transcript of speech delivered at Rice University, September 12, 1962, https://er.jsc.nasa.gov/seh/ricetalk.htm.

2. Hellen Keller, *Let Us Have Faith* (Garden City, NY: Doubleday, 1940), 50, 51.

3. Joan Guntzelman, *God Knows You're Grieving: Things to Do to Help You Through* (Notre Dame, IN: Sorin Books, 2001), 88–89.

4. Francis, *Evangelii gaudium* (November 24, 2013), n. 44.

5. Edward Everett Hale, cited in *A Year of Beautiful Thoughts*, ed. Jeanie A. B. Greenough (New York: Thomas Y. Crowell, 1902), 172.

Chapter 2

Who Am I Now?

We can draw inspiration from the lives of others who lived with a chronic condition. One example is an illustrious author who adjusted well to the limitations of her disease. Flannery O'Connor was the only child of Edward and Regina O'Connor. She was born in Savannah, Georgia, on March 24, 1925. Her father was diagnosed with systemic lupus erythematosus, an incurable autoimmune disease, in 1939. In 1940, as a result of her father's disease, they moved to their family farm, Andalusia, near Milledgeville, Georgia, which is now a museum dedicated to O'Connor's work. Her father died there in 1941 from the effects of lupus.

O'Connor earned a bachelor's of arts in social sciences and a masters's of fine arts in creative writing. Her writings reveal her quirky sense of humor, an uncanny grasp of the nuances of human behavior, literary irony, and a penchant for satire and comedy. In December 1950, she fell ill and was diagnosed with lupus like her father. Although she was expected to live for five years, she lived for fourteen. In 1959, she moved in with her mother at Andalusia and lived there until her death. During that time, she made lecture trips and visited friends, minding her physical limitations. When her mobility became limited by lupus, she used crutches. She spent her mornings writing and afternoons tending to her peacocks and other exotic birds. She also maintained a wide correspondence with friends and others who wrote to discuss her stories. She received many visitors who sought her advice on literary and spiritual matters.

Her stories reflected her concern for her fellow human beings, especially in the South. She received an honorary doctor of letters from Smith College in 1963. She is considered one of the greatest fiction writers of the twentieth century. During her life, O'Connor gave lectures on literature and faith, received numerous awards, and produced a significant number of cartoons, book reviews, essays, short stories, occasional poems, and two novels. Her texts usually took place in the South and involved morally flawed characters and disturbing themes, such as racism and poverty. Many of her short stories have been published in major anthologies, including *The Best American Short Stories*. She died from lupus complications on August 3, 1964. At the time of her death, the *Atlanta Journal-Constitution* noted that O'Connor's "deep spirituality qualified her to speak with a forcefulness not often matched in American literature"[1] In 2002, she was inducted as a charter member of the Georgia Writers Hall of Fame. In 2015, the US Postal Service honored her with a new postage stamp in their literary arts series.

Each one of us has a perception of his or her personal identity, those ways in which we think about ourselves or describe who we are. Positive stories like Flannery O'Connor's contribute to a positive identity concerning ourselves.

Who Am I Now?

Negative stories about pain and endless problems have the opposite effect. Positive aspects of our identity are strengthened by diligence and determination, and they lead to a satisfying and rewarding self-image.

However, identities can change over time. We pass through our adolescence, our student days, and our working years. As we get older, we may lose dearly held identities from key roles we play, such as spouse, nurturer, or provider, and gain identities that challenge us in different ways through disability, old age, or confinement. Over time we think and feel about ourselves in different ways. Maturity elevates us above peer pressure, popular trends, and physical aspects of ourselves and supports our unique identity, deeply held values, and heartfelt beliefs. Serious health issues can distance us from petty self-centeredness, social status, and other trivialities, and they can even bring our attention to kindness toward others, social responsibility, and stability found in renewed wholesomeness.

A father once played a game with his three children. He asked them, "If you could be anybody on Earth, who would you be?" One of the girls said, "I want to be Supergirl." The other daughter said she wanted to be Katniss Everdeen. The boy did not say a word. The father asked him, "Who would you like to be?" "I would like to be me," said the boy. "Why do you want to be you?" the father asked. "I like me," the boy responded. That was a fine response. That boy was more settled than his siblings. He did not want to be anyone else. He was at peace with himself.

Living with or through a major infirmity affects our identity. The quality of the effect is as unique as the identity of the person. From major to minor, it will influence one's sense of well-being and one's relationships with others. It takes brutal honesty to face the realities of a significant ailment. During diagnostic tests and treatments, our disease may be at the top of our identity list. When we finish our treatments and learn more about our type of disease, this label can become less significant for our concept of self. Even if we have a serious disease, we can still say yes to life. Poor health can move us to let go of the self we were used to in order to embrace a better self.

Reevaluating the Indicators of Self-Worth

In our society, body image is part of our identity and significantly affects our quality of life. Judging by the booming antiaging industry, most people are concerned about being attractive, some taking it to extremes. Whether we have a chronic condition or not, how many of us are satisfied with our body image? The majority of us would probably say "not me." This is especially true when undergoing treatment, which can alter a person's body. Many changes can be temporary. For example, common side effects of cancer therapy include hair loss, weight change, radiation skin burns, mouth sores, changes in hormones, or dry and cracked skin. Some changes are permanent, such as surgical scarring, amputation, mastectomy, or an ostomy. How we see our external wounds depends not on what we see, but on how we perceive what we see. Wounds can range in meaning, from something that is repulsive to something that is a sign of courage.

How a person's body is affected by disease and its treatments varies depending on the individual and the type of disease. Whatever the change, it can make us feel less mascu-

Who Am I Now?

line or less feminine, less vital, or more emotionally sensitive. We may feel estranged, like we don't fit in anymore, are less capable, or are not able to provide for or protect our family. Side effects may make us feel worse than the disease itself. There are several things we can do to counteract this train of thought when chemotherapy, radiation, or other long-term treatments seem endless. We can reward ourselves after the day's treatment, think about what we are going to do after the last appointment, list the positive elements of our journey, or focus on the good things that happened during the month. We can talk to a friend or participate in a group. Social, moral, and spiritual supports are great assets when enduring any serious experience. Martin Luther King Jr. wrote, "My personal trials have also taught me the value of unmerited suffering. As my sufferings mounted I soon realized that there were two ways that I could respond to my situation: either to react with bitterness or seek to transform the suffering into a creative force. ... If only to save myself from bitterness, I have attempted to see my personal ordeals as an opportunity to transform myself and heal the people involved in the tragic situation which now obtains. I have lived these last few years with the conviction that unearned suffering is redemptive."[2]

Good looks do not have first place on the list of what is beautiful. We must see beyond the physical to the beauty of the person within. Intangible personal qualities are a crucial part of being attractive. Perhaps we are not as aware of them as we should be. They can be like a bouquet of beautiful flowers: daisies for a delightful sense of humor, daffodils for common sense, violets for charm, marigolds for good manners, hyacinths for trustworthiness, roses for a certain sweetness, and magnolias for clear thinking. These internal traits are more precious than our external anatomy. A health problem can provide the opportunity to learn new things about ourselves as well as to learn new skills and hobbies. Learning something new will always trump physical appearance as a source of positive self-image. We may no longer be able to participate in high-impact activities or take pride in our physical prowess. However, crafts that develop from woodworking, sewing, painting, needlepoint, or ceramics can be more rewarding by giving us a new sense of pride and accomplishment. We can keep the results or, better still, give them as gifts. And wouldn't it be good for the environment to learn how to fix something instead of disposing of it and buying something new? We should also never forget the beauty of the mind, heart, and soul. Gaining knowledge, helping others, and nurturing faith can be sound supports for self-worth and more rewarding than compliments regarding our appearance.

Hope Alive in All Situations

The energy that keeps us moving on a journey with a chronic disease is hope, which is much more than wishful thinking or optimism. Anchored in divine providence, it is an inner buoyancy of the heart that keeps troubling circumstances in check. When we are going through hard times, we may not be completely focused on hope, because it is hidden by the dark clouds of health concerns. However, it lies in the depths of the heart, and when we become conscious of that, we can transcend the troubles of the day, staying stable and alert, regardless of how things turn out. Because hope stems from faith, it goes beyond the boundaries of the mind and the confines of the here and now. Hope flows from striving to see ourselves and those around us through the eyes of God and to recognize his love at work. This concerns us as well. Rev. Henry Melville wrote (in a quote often misattributed to Herman Melville) that hope "is the struggle of the soul, breaking loose from what is perishable and attesting to her eternity."[3]

Hope is like a strong thread that is woven throughout the fabric of life. It is not simply a darning thread used to mend patches of difficulties with a few cheery words or scattered good deeds. Hope sustains a lifelong belief that something better can be attained. When dealing with a long-term disease, we may discover surprising new things concerning our identity. We may be more courageous than we ever thought. We may discover a refreshing resiliency. In his *Summa theologiae*, St. Thomas Aquinas said that hope is an activity concerned with a future good that is difficult but possible to accomplish with the help of God (II-II.17.1 corpus). Hope puts all health concerns in the hands of God with confidence that he will not drop them. Maintaining hope when a situation appears to be hopeless keeps us moving ahead.

People who have chronic conditions will gaze upon barren trees and walk on icy roads on their journey. There will be times when life seems bleak like an endless cold winter. We may even think that our spiritual practices are useless, a waste of time with no merit. Sr. Wendy Beckett responds, "Body and soul may feel we are wasting our time. Hope smiles and ignores them."[4] Hope always takes us beyond the immediacy of pain and sorrow in the present and into the possibilities of the future:

> The earth lies cold and dark,
> and blackened trees
> are sentinels of silhouetted

loneliness against the bleak,
stark nakedness of day.
Unwarmed, unwelcome,
I make my way through
landscape damp and chill:
even the birds are silent;
even the trees are still!
I listen to my heavy step:
I hear no other thing,
'Til out of grey curtained distance,
a bluebird and chickadee sing![5]

Self-Confidence, a Strong and Sturdy Attribute

A sound identity is rooted in self-confidence, which can take a real beating from the many physical and emotional changes that come with managing health concerns. We experience periods of apathy, confusion, uncertainty, vacillations, and other unsavory feelings. These can be expected because we need time to adjust to the changes of a chronic disease and its related events that have a negative effect on our self-confidence. We worry about the results of an upcoming diagnostic test, are overly anxious about a visit with our doctor, or dread the side effects of prescriptions. We feel utterly out of control. However, our self-confidence can get a positive boost when we believe we are not alone in our struggles. Many people care about our well-being, even those whom we do not know, like a friend of a friend.

Underneath all our strife, we are still loveable, gifted, and valuable persons. Self-confidence is strengthened when we acknowledge that the source of our giftedness comes from God. Disease reminds us that life involves struggle and difficulties, but they can be managed with compassion and goodness. Good choices are made after consulting with learned people and listening at prayer. Mature decision-making discerns the components of a choice in the context of eternity and a life well-lived.

Whether we have a chronic condition or not, we are all players on the human stage. Disease touches everyone in some way, and each of us can do something—from annually donating to a society dedicated to a specific disease to visiting a homebound acquaintance or volunteering at a local foundation. One role of people of who have a long-term disease is that of teacher, and what we learn can inspire new ideas for one of the many aspects of health care. Samuel Johnson wrote, "Self-confidence is the first requisite to great undertakings."[6] Small undertakings can become great institutions. Strength is associated with an old interpretation of confidence, which John Dewey defines as "directness and courage in meeting the facts of life, trusting them to bring instruction and support to a developing self."[7]

In his first inaugural address, declaring war on the Great Depression, President Franklin Roosevelt said that confidence "thrives only on honesty, on honor, on the sacredness of obligations, on faithful protection, on unselfish performance; without them it cannot live."[8] When we live these words, we connect with our true selves. No disease, person, or society can make us feel inferior or fearful without our consent. We need not find our genuine identity in a diagnosis, a negative childhood event, or social trends. Other people's thoughts or opinions are not our reality, especially when they concern grim data. Charles Stanley said that fear "stifles thinking and snuffs out creativity. [It] causes tension in the body, which often leads to temporary emotional paralysis or a failure to act."[9] Lost opportunities erode confidence: "You gain strength, courage, and confidence by every experience in which you really stop to look fear in the face. You are able to say to yourself, 'I lived through this horror. I can take the next thing that comes along.'"[10]

Living with a chronic condition gives us many opportunities to look fear in the face. Believing in ourselves, our convictions, and our abilities; trusting in God; and maintaining a hopeful optimism help us to overcome fear. People can have more confidence in us if they see we understand and can communicate the various aspects of their diseases. They may also have confidence in us because they see the gifts and talents in us that we do not see or because they admire our bravery and tenacity in times of trial.

Self-Knowledge, a Primary Necessity

Self-knowledge, which is a lifelong endeavor that gives us insights into our true selves, is essential for self-identity. It is the quality that keeps suffering in perspective. Sometimes suffering can shake us out of a self-destructive, complacent, or superficial lifestyle. Suffering, under the umbrella of self-knowledge, can still the restlessness in our hearts and the questions in our minds and replace them with inner peace. Self-knowledge teaches us not to blame ourselves, others, or God for suffering, which comes from the evil in humanity and natural causes. Self-knowledge strengthens faltering faith by providing courage that takes us beyond negative or ambivalent feelings or hesitations. When we do not know what lies

Who Am I Now?

ahead, courage stands us up on our feet and gives us the shove we need to move forward.

Since we rely so much on others on our journey through chronic disease, we learn the value of humility. We feel humble when people do things for us that we were previously able to do ourselves. Humility is more than a feeling. It is a vital component of self-knowledge as well as a lifelong virtue that ensures a sound identity. At its highest level, this virtue imparts the desire to see ourselves as we stand before God. Alive within us, it is like a quiet, ever-present warm light, devoid of grandeur or fuss, yet a fire full of unobtrusive wisdom, a good portion of which is gleaned on the trail of life. Chronic disorders can make us become more attentive to the consequences of certain behaviors and to what is beneficial and what is harmful to us. Humility helps us to strive, in the best way possible, to do what seems to be right as we manage the challenges of less-than-optimal health. As we live with humility, we learn to get out of our own way, keep our chronic condition in its rightful place, and maintain a clear-minded, childlike confidence in God: "Lay all care for the future, confidently, in God's hands, and allow yourself to be led by him entirely, as a child would. Then you can be sure not to lose your way."[11]

It is possible to deepen a positive self-identity and self-knowledge after we reflect on what we gained from walking through or with difficulties. We realize it has given us an inner strength, greater resilience, and a more compassionate outlook. Flannery O'Connor said that her lupus was "more instructive than a long trip to Europe."[12] People with significant health issues can give back in ways they never expected.

Courage through Chronic Disease

After her cancer treatment, Sally Jo, a licensed cosmetologist, helped women with cancer by teaching them how to apply makeup and care for their hair, nails, and skin. She found this more rewarding than working with her pre-cancer customers. Barbara, a hair stylist who experienced cancer, became a specialist in designing and fitting wigs for patients with hair loss. Although we should use the adage "never say never" sparingly when speaking about participating in new activities or developing new skills, physical challenges can give us a new purpose or even a new calling in life. After his presidency, when he was in his sixties, Ulysses S. Grant developed throat cancer. During this period, he wrote his memoir, which became a best-selling book on the Civil War.

Benedetta Bianchi Porro was born in Forli, Italy, on August 8, 1936. An intelligent and happy child, she wrote, "The universe is enchanting! It is great to be alive."[13] When she was a teenager, she began to lose her hearing. However, she entered medical school, read the lips of her professors, and excelled in her studies. After five years of medical training, just one year short of earning her degree, she was forced to end her studies after diagnosing herself with von Recklinghausen's disease, a neurological condition that would ultimately cause her to lose all five of her senses, leaving her paralyzed and able to move only one hand. Her suffering threatened to plunge her into despair. From her seventh-floor apartment, Benedetta wrote to a friend, "There are times that I would like to throw myself out the window."[14] On a trip to Lourdes, she had an interior healing and said, "I am aware more than ever of the richness of my condition and I don't desire anything but to continue in it."[15] She knew the value of her life and became a kind of doctor of the soul to those who visited her. She was strengthened by the love of Jesus. In the end, Benedetta was able to write, "I do not lack hope. I know that at the end of the road, Jesus is waiting for me. ... My days are not easy. They are hard. But sweet because Jesus is with me."[16] She went home to the Lord on January 23, 1964.

Gratitude, a Song from the Heart

We read in the Gospel according to Luke,

> On the way to Jerusalem he was passing along between Samaria and Galilee. And as he entered a village, he was met by ten lepers, who stood at a distance and lifted up their voices and said, "Jesus, Master, have mercy on us." When he saw them he said to them, "Go and show yourselves to the priests." And as they went they were cleansed. Then one of them, when he saw that he was healed, turned back, praising God with a loud voice; and he fell on his face at Jesus' feet, giving him thanks. Now he was a Samaritan. Then said Jesus, "Were not ten cleansed? Where are the nine? Was no one found to return and give praise to God except this foreigner?" And he said to him, "Rise and go your way; your faith has made you well" (17:11–19).

Persons who have a long-term disease, can be grateful for many things, the greatest of which is life. They have learned to be grateful for complex things and common activities of daily living, like eating, sleeping, and walking, that may have been problematic during treatment. Gratitude is the baseline of a sound identity. Chronic health problems can broaden our practice of gratitude because daily tasks are no longer taken for granted. We may have considered our gratitude only once a year on Thanksgiving Day, but now we are grateful for the good and not-so-good things that happen to us each day.

An elderly woman had two large pots hung on the ends of a pole that she carried across her shoulders. One of the pots had a crack in it, while the other pot was perfect. At the end of the long walk from the stream to the house, the cracked pot arrived only half full. Each day for two years, the woman would bring home only one-and-a-half pots of water. The perfect pot was proud of its accomplishments. The cracked pot was ashamed of its imperfection and miserable because it could do only half of what it had been made to do. After two years, it spoke to the woman by the stream: "I am ashamed of myself because this crack in my side causes water to leak out all the way back to your house." The old woman smiled, "Did you notice that there are flowers on your side of the path but not on the other side? That is because I have always known about your flaw, so I planted flower seeds on your side of the path, and every day on our walk back, you watered them. For two years, I have been able to pick these beautiful flowers to decorate the table. Without you being just the way you are, there would not be this beauty to grace my house." Chronic disease cracks our earthen vessels. How do we react to those cracks? Do we look at them with dark stares, or do we see the light that shines from them? When we see this light, we are grateful. Gratitude reveals that the light from our cracks can nurture others. Indeed, grace can have strange wrappings.

Gratitude is an interior and exterior experience. An internal interpretation is to maintain a grateful heart that recognizes all gifts received. This is followed by an external expression of words or deeds that acknowledges and gives thanks to the giver of a gift. Some type of appreciation is said or written. We can remember when our mothers reminded us to write thank-you notes for our gifts. That advice is as good now as it was then. When it is appropriate, some token of gratitude is extended for what has been freely given by the donor. If we are invited to a dinner at a friend's home, we thank her for the invitation and bring her flowers. Gratitude is a beautiful practice because it is not hampered by negative traits. It is an art form that requires cultivation by use. We learn to embrace the moment, savor its joy, and affirm the goodness in others.

Psychological studies have found a positive correlation between gratitude and happiness. The practice of being a grateful person develops from conscious choices. It is a decision more than a feeling. It can be a beautiful, spontaneous remark as well as an antidote that dilutes the effects of evil in our society. During difficulties we focus on what went right rather than what went wrong. Gratitude opens a door so that we can see beauty in places where we never expected to find it, even in an examination room. We give thanks for things we took for granted. The morning alarm reminds us to be grateful for another day. Income tax reminds us that we have a job and money is coming in. Squabbling offspring remind us we have children to love.

Being thankful goes beyond being polite or saying something that is expected of us. A habit of gratitude matures us. It is a grace that comes from the heart. If we reflect upon our lives, we see the effects of gratitude when we choose to help not hurt; to remedy not reveal; to elevate not diminish; to illuminate not darken. These traits can come to the forefront as we meet people during our journey of chronic disease. The strong threads of gratitude are unassuming and inconspicuous, weaving their way into the hearts of fellow sojourners and into the fabric of the passing days. In muted shades, a grateful heart gives joy to the downhearted, rest to those who are weary, and quiet to those who are too busy. Unexpected graces help us to be loving, patient, gentle, tender, and ever grateful for daily gifts, wherever we are.

Our self-identity is more than what we perceive. Perceptions of reality can bind or free us. Each person's description of us will be different. In the long run, we are responsible for what we think, what we do, and how we treat others. We strive to be empathetic in the way described by Atticus Finch in *To Kill a Mockingbird*: "You never really understand a person until you consider things from his point of view, until you climb into his skin and walk around in it."[17] To immerse oneself in humanity is to enter into its pain, brokenness, confusion, and anguish. Living with a chronic disease makes us more aware of these conditions. In spite of the suffering we experience and observe, we are grateful for life. Gratitude is threefold: It is the virtue that makes us aware of the gifts we receive each day. It moves us to respond to these gifts by developing them, using them well, and putting them at the service of others. And, finally, it makes us more appreciative of the generosity of God. This is expressed beautifully in the hymn "We Plough the Fields, and Scatter":

> We thank you then, dear Father.
> For all things bright and good.
> The seedtime and the harvest,
> Our life, our health, our food.

Who Am I Now?

And all that we can offer,
Your boundless love imparts.
The gifts to you most pleasing
Are humble, thankful hearts.

Notes

1. Cited in Sarah Gordon, "Flannery O'Connor," *New Georgia Encyclopedia*, updated April 5, 2021, https://www.georgiaencyclopedia.org/articles/arts-culture/flannery-oconnor-1925-1964/.

2. Martin Luther King Jr., "Suffering and Faith," *Transcript of speech delivered in Chicago*, April 27, 1960, https://kinginstitute.stanford.edu/king-papers/documents/suffering-and-faith

3. Henry Melville, "The Advantage of State Expectation," in *Sermons*, vol. 1, ed. C.P. M'Ilvaine (New York: Stanford and Swords, 1850), 113.

4. Wendy Beckett, *Sister Wendy on Prayer* (New York: Harmony Books, 2006), 120.

5. This poem comes from a holy card from the Carmelite Monastery in Terre Haute, Indiana. Monastery website: https://heartsawake.org/index.php.

6. George Birkbeck Hill, *Wit and Wisdom of Samuel Johnson* (Oxford: Clarendon Press, 1888), 258.

7. John Dewey, *Human Nature and Conduct: An Introduction to Social Psychology* (New York: Henry Holt, 1922), 139.

8. Franklin D. Roosevelt, "First Inaugural Address," transcript of speech delivered March 4, 1933, https://avalon.law.yale.edu/20th_century/froos1.asp.

9. Charles Stanley, *Can You Still Trust God? What Happens When You Choose to Believe* (Nashville: Nelson Books, 2021), 162.

10. Eleanor Roosevelt, *You Learn by Living: Eleven Keys for a More Fulfilling Life* (Louisville, KY: Westminster John Knox Press, 1960), 29.

11. Edith Stein, Letter to Ruth Kantorowitz, in *Self-Portrait in Letters*, 1916–1942, trans. Josephine Koeppel (Washington, DC: ICS Publications, 1934), n. 181.

12. Flannery O'Connor, "Letter to A (June 28, 1956)," in *The Habit of Being*, ed. Sally Fitzgerald (New York: Farrar, Straus, and Giroux, 1988), 163.

13. Benedetta Bianchi Porro, cited in Liz Kelly, "She Held Jesus in Her Palm: Meet Blessed Benedetta," Catholic Spirit, September 25, 2019, https://thecatholicspirit.com/commentary/your-heart-his-home/she-held-jesus-in-her-palm-meet-blessed-benedetta/.

14. Benedetta Bianchi Porro, cited in Antoine Marie, *Letter to Friends of the Abbey of Saint-Joseph de Clairval*, January 21, 2011, https://www.clairval.com/index.php/en/letter/?id=2190111.

15. Porro, cited in Liz Kelly, "She Held Jesus in Her Palm."

16. Porro, cited in Antoine Marie, *Letter to Friends*.

17. Harper Lee, *To Kill a Mockingbird*, 40th anniversary ed. (New York: HarperCollins Books, 1960), 33.

Chapter 3

Aspects of Care

It is not uncommon for the expression of caring love to change as the years pass. A dramatic example is the life of Rose Hawthorne Lathrop. She was born in Lenox, Massachusetts, in 1851 but spent her childhood years in Liverpool, England, because her father, Nathaniel Hawthorne, was the US counsel there. She came home to Concord, Massachusetts, in 1860. Rose married George Parsons Lathrop when she was twenty, and they settled in Boston. George worked at the *Atlantic Monthly*, and Rose established her reputation as a writer by publishing short stories and poems. After five years, a son, Francis Hawthorne Lathrop, was born, but he died of diphtheria when he was only five years old.

Rose and George were received into the Catholic Church in 1891, ten years after their son's death. When George developed problems with "intemperance," he could no longer hold a job, and his and Rose's marriage became intolerable. With her confessor's authorization, Rose began to live by herself, took nurse's training, and started to work with patients suffering from incurable cancer. This was a heartbreaking ministry to which she devoted the rest of her life. After George's death in 1898, Rose became a Dominican sister and, with other like-minded women, established the Dominican Congregation of St. Rose of Lima, also known as the Servants of Relief for Incurable Cancer. She was the order's first mother superior and took the name Mother Mary Alphonsa. Their first center for cancer patients was established in Hawthorne, New York, where she spent the rest of her years. She died there in 1936.

Rose was a lady of culture, education, and social status who put on an apron and used her gifts to serve Christ's poor. She lived among the needy, begged for them, and established several homes where they could live their final days in dignity, ease, cleanliness, and peace. There was no class system among the residents and religious sisters. The sisters were true servants, and the residents were recipients of their care and concern. The sisters and their mission continue today.

To serve is an act of love. Caregiving is composed of innumerable acts that make up the art of love, which is more difficult and more challenging than other forms of art, such as painting nature scenes, composing a sonata, sculpting a statue, or writing a book. Like no other art form, caregiving has unique burdens and rewards because the caregiver is devoted to serving another. There is great value in giving care because it is a contribution to the good of humankind and an expression of God's love.

To assume responsibility for someone who has multiple daily living needs takes a great deal of courage. Even though caregivers do not know what predicaments wait on the roadside, or what concerns lie around the corner, they pick up the reins and move forward. Moreover, assuming the role of caregiver can dramatically alter a person's personal life and daily routine, and he or she relinquishes much of their independence with this new duty. Nevertheless, caregiving can be a call to a love we didn't know was possible:

> At a workshop several years ago, a woman shared this story: She was the mother of four children and, while they were all still young, at home, in school, her father, already a widower, suffered a stroke that left him severely debilitated. He was unable to take care of himself and needed assistance.
>
> Being the dutiful daughter, she had him move in with her own family, at great inconvenience to her husband and children. So many of their family routines had to be adjusted and rearranged to accommodate her dad's presence. Their life changed radically.
>
> At a point, her father's condition deteriorated to the point where she had to take him to a hospice where he could receive full-time care. But, even then, she still needed to visit him daily, often having to take one or more of her children with her. This went on for seven years. Daily, she and one or other of her children would have to go and spend some time with her father.
>
> During those years, many times, in large and small ways, she apologized to her husband and children for the inconvenience this was causing them. Eventually her father died. Several years after the funeral her eldest son, now in college, said to her: "You know, Mum, all those years that we had to arrange our lives so much around Grandpa and his illness—that was really a precious time. That was a great gift to our family!"[1]

Caregiving has different stages: acute care, rehab care, and palliative care. There are different techniques and ways of caring in each phase. To encourage or caution, praise or correct, be assertive or receptive will be different within each area. The patient should decide when help is needed and avoid being waited on. There may be a difference between the patient's and caregiver's perception of the patient's needs. Although it is easier to dress a patient rather than wait while he is slowly trying to dress himself, to wait encourages the patient to repossess this daily task. The patient should have as much control as he is able to handle. Another positive note is to avoid thinking of a setback (e.g., no longer being able to walk to the bathroom) as a loss of control but rather as a change of strategy. This parallels using non-judgmental terms, such as referring to a paralyzed arm as the "involved arm" instead of a "bad arm."

The following sections provide practical guidance for these different aspects of caregiving. Some occur at a specific stage, and others persist throughout the entire continuum, perhaps being easier or more difficult at different times. While reading through these strategies, reflect on Ralph Waldo Emerson's meditation for caregivers: "This is my wish for you: Comfort on difficult days, smiles when sadness intrudes, rainbows to follow the clouds, laughter to kiss your lips, sunsets to warm your heart, hugs when spirits sag, beauty for your eyes to see, friendships to brighten your being, faith so that you can believe, confidence for when you doubt, courage to know yourself, patience to accept the truth, love to complete your life."[2]

Do Not Ignore Self-Care

A caregiver, first and foremost, needs to take care of herself.[3] She cannot neglect her own health and personal needs or put them on the back burner. Compromising physical, mental, or spiritual health weakens her capacity to respond to her patient's needs. Self-care includes basics, such as good eating habits, suitable weight, regular exercise, emotional stability, spiritual practices, appropriate medications, and adequate sleep. She should also be aware of when she is experiencing burnout.

Assign Duties to Appropriate People

A caregiver can be expected to perform a broad spectrum of duties, and it is necessary to put together a list of specific responsibilities. These include knowing the patient's medical history, cleaning house, providing transportation, providing encouragement, and emptying drains. The list goes on and leaves one breathless.

When a caregiver begins her service, her specific duties should include realistic and clearly defined guidelines regarding daily responsibilities and patient behavior. This avoids unrealistic demands or expectations, and a caregiver skill is to learn how to appropriately say no when asked to go beyond what she is expected to do or to perform tasks beyond her capabilities. A harmful hallmark of our society is the "busy bee syndrome." Og Mandino tells us, "The weakest living creature, by concentrating his powers on a single object, can accomplish good results while the strongest, by dispersing his effort over many chores, may fail to accomplish anything. Drops of water, by continually falling, hone their passage through the hardest of rocks but the hasty torrent rushes over it with hideous uproar and leaves no trace behind."[4]

A caregiver cannot be responsible for everything. She needs to enlist the help of family and friends. Sometimes adult children can be better at one type of care, spouses at another type of care, and friends at yet another type of care. It would be advantageous to create a team of volunteers composed of family, friends, church members, and neighbors. If people want to help, they should be specific regarding what they would like to do. "How can I help?" is a well-meaning question, but a better question is directed to a task and when it can be done. A calendar showing who will be doing what, on what day, and at what time would be helpful: bringing dinner over on two specific days of the week, gardening on Saturday, shopping on Monday, laundry on Tuesday, house cleaning on Wednesday, and taking out the trash on Friday. Support can also come in the form of gift certificates for groceries, cleaning services, manicures, and so forth.

Often people serve as caregivers and do not even realize it. Their example shows that caregiving duties do not have to be burdensome. Once a week for about three years, Tina and her husband Jerry have been delivering Meals on Wheels to a high-rise apartment building for low-income seniors. They never stopped, even during the pandemic. Most of the residents have chronic conditions and little family support. Tina and Jerry serve just by providing one more opportunity to check on the seniors and make sure they are doing okay. If there is a need, Jerry or Tina will call the Meals on Wheels office, and someone there will follow up. Alice's sister-in-law has early signs of dementia and multiple other chronic conditions. Her brother works during the week driving a city bus. When her sister-in-law feels up to it, Alice goes over for an afternoon, and they play dominoes. Alice usually must remind her of the rules about every five minutes, but they laugh and talk and have a wonderful time.

Despite all the help that can be given by family and friends, many people are prone to offer well-intentioned but inappropriate advice. It is prudent for the caregiver to defer to health care professionals who know the person for whom she is caring. If well-meaning suggestions and opinions from others cause additional confusion and stress, the caregiver can thank the person and let the information go in one ear and out the other. Another challenge is dealing with the patient's personal relationships. No doubt, there will be friends and relatives who avoid the patient after his diagnosis. They no longer visit or make direct contact by phone or e-mail. This is more common than not. These people may never have had contact with anyone who has had a serious disease, they don't know how to deal with it, or they fear "catching" it. They do not know what to say or what to do. This is all disappointing, but it is best to keep good thoughts about these people because they are battling their own demons. People should be discouraged from visiting if they have long, sad faces; are insensitive; ask intrusive questions; predict gloomy prospects; or tell dismal stories. If a positive environment is prevalent, it will help dilute the negative habits of people and even reveal threads of humor in them.

Promote Optimism in the Relationship

A good quality of the caregiver is to maintain a stable, upbeat, positive orientation while at work. This is quite challenging, but it is necessary for the well-being of the patient. A caregiver will not be able to lift her patient's spirits if she is down in the dumps. She can strive to be upbeat as she does her best to love, care, and comfort the patient. How a caregiver faces her patient's difficulties reflects how she faces her own. Her thoughts about life, death, health, disease, religion, and God all affect, in greater or lesser degrees, how she cares for another. A caregiver has her own troubles that cause her concern. However, worrying about those while taking care of a patient burdens that care with additional weight.

Serious disease is a return to *terra firma*. Life can get very basic for people who are chronically ill, and another task of optimistic caregiving is keeping the patient in a current time frame. Time is limited, and everybody should try to do their best with the time they have left. To concentrate on real needs rather than mere wants and to live not in the regrets of the past or dreams of the future, but in the beauty and blessings of today, are essential. Helen Keller wrote, "When one door of happiness closes, another opens; but often we look so long at the closed door that we do not see the one which has been opened for us."[5] It is fitting for the patient to muse about happiness in the past as long as the patient does not stay there. When that seems likely, the caregiver gently reminds the patient that indeed, there are doors of happiness waiting to be opened today. Life is temporary and unpredictable, but it is precious.

Listen to the Patient's Perspective

Listening is an art. In order to practice it, the caregiver cannot be entrenched in her own views, which prevent her from listening or from receiving constructive feedback. No one wants to be an incorrigible caregiver. To listen with the ears of the heart requires effort, attention, and concentration.

Aspects of Care

It comes from a quiet space within. The quiet is a reminder not to interrupt when being told something, not to think about responses when listening, or not to respond with a similar situation. The quiet space helps to listen to what is said, as well as to what is not said, in order to be sensitive to unexpressed feelings. To stay in tune with what is said puts aside one's own agenda, insights, and unsought advice.

A caregiver is a companion and listener more than a strategic advisor. She avoids jumping in with her corrections, judgments, or criticisms. She remembers that she is different from the individual for whom she is caring. She needs to think twice about saying things that are meaningful to her but may not be of value to the person to whom she is giving care. A few encouraging words may gently persuade the patient to share his feelings or prioritize what activities are most important. If this happens, listen and let the patient talk without pressing issues. Some people are very private, and others like to talk about what they are going through. The caregiver listens not so much to respond, but to understand what the patient is thinking. She might ask questions to clarify or add to what the patient is saying. The caregiver is realistic and flexible regarding when the patient wants to talk, be quiet, or be alone.

Moreover, the caregiver acknowledges and validates the patient's feelings of the day, which may be ever-changing: anger, joy, depression, elation, sadness, happiness, confusion, or understanding. Even though the caregiver shares a patient's joy and sorrow, she respects his privacy. This means that outside of medical concerns, she does not ask intrusive questions. She strives to meet her patient where he is and not where she wants him to be. Finally, sometimes actions can speak louder than words. Just holding the patient's hand, resting a hand on his shoulder, or giving him a foot massage can be comforting beyond words.

Silence it as the heart of listening: "Learn to get in touch with silence within yourself and know that everything in this life has a purpose. There are no mistakes, no coincidences; all events are blessings given to us to learn from."[6] Silence is more than the absence of words, noise, distractions, or diversions. It opens the way to greater tolerance, respect, good humor, dignity, gentleness, prayer, and connection with God. We are reminded of the nursery rhyme: "A wise old owl sat in an oak. The more he heard the less he spoke. The less he spoke the more he heard. Why can't we all be like that bird?"

Focus on the Person, Not the Disease

Treating the patient as a person with many attributes is more affirming than treating him as sick and in need of help. Attending to activities that are not related to chronic disease acknowledges a life of integration. A sick patient is a person of many parts that can be more real than the sickness. The caregiver strives to walk the line that is strong but not overpowering, that is able to extend empathy but refrains from pity, that is firm and tactful but not condescending or patronizing, and that remains realistic but not discouraging.

If the caregiver gives all her attention to fixing that which is broken or doing chores, she needs to slow down and consider the mutuality of care. Giving care is not unilateral. Instead of running around in a perpetual hurry to get things done, the caregiver sits down and is truly present to the patient. They can discuss how to do this or that activity better, or other things that are unrelated to the chronic disease or the care it requires. Loving service should not become a mechanical or chaotic routine. If a caregiver sits quietly near her patient, she can give him an opportunity to share a story or something that has been troubling him. While sitting, the caregiver can be like a candle with a still flame of hope, a quiet light of faith, and a warm embrace of love.

Even though homebound patients can be uncomfortable or embarrassed when they need help with personal care, they realize this is in the job description of caregivers, and they are used to it. Caregivers do not think about the need to be needed, because it is obvious. Conversely, each person, including those who are debilitated, have a basic desire to be needed. How can a person meet the need to be needed when he is a homebound patient?

There are ways of giving back to those who give care. Homebound patients can express their appreciation for little things like the scent of fragrant soap, a bird's song, a beautiful flower, the taste of a homemade muffin, or the touch of a warm hand. They can gratefully acknowledge the things people do for them, such as cleaning the kitchen, watering the plants, or folding the laundry. A sincere thank you is like balm on the heart. Patients can use the talents and gifts they still have as much as they can. Every little bit helps. If they can no longer do something they enjoyed, like baking a pie or building a birdhouse, they can instruct others how to do it. Instead of fixing a leak in the faucet themselves, they can tell another member of the household how to do it. They can be kind and say caring and supportive things, even though at times they do not feel like being kind. They do their best not to complain and especially not to whine about being a burden. When we feel inclined to moan and groan about our situation, we can do so to God. He will understand completely.

A positive attitude will motivate homebound patients to engage in cognitive challenges that stretch their intellect. They can do crossword puzzles, and when the answer remains a mystery, they can ask the caregiver. It has been said that the best moments of life happen when your mind is stretched to accomplish something worthwhile. Working on a task that challenges our ability to think is good mental exercise. Memorizing data gives us a sense of accomplishment and a reason to quiz the caregiver. We can learn 1 Corinthians 13, ten people who won the Nobel Prize, all the lines from a favorite old song, the twelve cranial nerves, the books of the New Testament, or the Gettysburg Address. The possibilities are endless.

Be a Patient Advocate

The most important duty of a caregiver is to be the patient's advocate, an intercessor for the patient who speaks for or takes action on behalf of his best interests. She can protect the patient from inappropriate visitors, unnecessary procedures, and problematic situations that occur during medical visits or hospitalizations. When dealing with troublesome events or unpleasant people, the caregiver must talk with the people involved using a calm, nonconfrontational, and respectful approach. Having the caregiver go to bat for the patient is comforting to him because he is coping with a serious chronic condition and needs someone who is reliable to keep watch, stand up for, or intervene when something is wrong or not understood.

This is especially notable at medical appointments. The patient may be scared, confused, anxious, exhausted, or intimidated. The caregiver maintains emotional stability and can report interim symptoms, ask pertinent questions, interpret correctly what the health care professional has to say, and clarify changes in daily routine. The caregiver can also tend to post-appointment details, such as filling and picking up prescriptions, making follow-up appointments, and addressing insurance issues. The caregiver is that extra pair of eyes and ears that pick up what a lone patient can miss and the voice that says things the patient may be too afraid or embarrassed to bring up. With caregiver accompaniment, the patient can have a greater feeling of security and confidence.

Be Prepared for Setbacks

Even though a caregiver has good intentions, she should be prepared for disappointments. Her suggestions may not be sought or taken seriously by the patient or his family. A patient's behavior may be rude, insulting, contrary, or unpredictable. The patient may be irritated by the caregiver and make no bones about letting her know it. To remain sane, the caregiver has to deflect negative behaviors like water off a duck's back. Let them go, be patient, and pray. If the patient is not motivated or is passive about his disease, advice from the caregiver may fall flat. Nagging, cajoling, or begging can build up the patient's resistance. The caregiver can gently try to lift the patient's spirits and quietly suggest having confidence in the health care team and in God. However, if nothing works, she can find comfort in prayer, rest in the heart of Jesus, and hope for a better day.

In Katherine Hume's novel *The Nun's Story*, one of the sister's advice to young nurses can provide encouragement to caregivers whose work seems unbearable:

Courage through Chronic Disease

All for Jesus, Sister William had said in the ward, pulling on the rubber gloves. Say it, my dear students, every time you are called upon for what seems an impossible task. Then you can do anything with serenity. It is a talisman phrase that takes away the disagreeable inherent in many nursing duties. Say it for the bedpans you carry, for the old incontinents you bathe, for those sputum cups of the tubercular. Tout pour Jésus, she said briskly as she bent to change a dressing foul with corruption. Gabrielle, Jeannine, Charlotte ... come closer and watch how I do this. You see how easy. All for Jesus ... This is no beggar's body picked up in the Rue des Radis. This is the body of Christ and this suppurating sore is one of His Wounds.[7]

There are layers within suffering that cannot be fixed. As much as a caregiver would like, she cannot solve all the patient's problems. Caring for others is a privilege rather than an obligation. Her regular presence and time demonstrates her tenacious fidelity and compassion. Compassion means "to suffer with." Her presence and her time, in good times and in bad, are signs that she is an authentic caregiver, an agent for her patient in partnership with her patient. We are all members of the human family. We are all weak and frail in some areas but strong and sturdy in others:

> God give me the serenity
> to accept the things I cannot change;
> courage to change the things I can;
> and the wisdom to know the difference.
> Living one day at a time;
> enjoying one moment at a time;

accepting hardships as the pathway to peace;
taking, as He did, this sinful world
as it is, not as I would have it;
trusting that He will make all things right
if I surrender to His will;
that I may be reasonably happy in this life
and supremely happy with Him
forever in the next.
Amen.

A chronic physical condition can be a teacher. As the patient's ability to control things slowly decreases, it becomes more apparent that no one has complete control. When personal defenses are released, we are able to rest in knowing that God is truly in control and that he doesn't give people diseases. Jesus said, "I am with you always, even unto the end of the world" (Matt. 28:20). There comes a time when we realize in our heads and in our hearts that we are truly in God's hands. The more we believe this, the more interior beauty we attain.

Notes

1. Ronald Rolheiser, "Of Elders, Character, Christ's Passion, and Blessing," reposted on Lifeissues, accessed August 29, 2022, https://www.lifeissues.net/writers/ron/ron_472.html.
2. Ralph Waldo Emerson, *Everyday Emerson: A Year of Wisdom* ed. Sam Torode, (New York. St. Martin's Press, 2022), June 6.
3. Caregiving is neither gender-specific nor gender-favored. Men and women are both called to this vocation with different gifts and skills but equal compassion. However, since the majority of caregivers are female, and for easier reading and a better flow of words, caregivers here will be referred to in the feminine.

4. Og Mandino, *The Greatest Salesman in the World*, part 2, The End of the Story (New York: Bantam Books, 1989), 115.

5. Helen Keller, *We Bereaved* (New York: Leslie Fulenwider, 1929), 23.

6. Elisabeth Kübler-Ross, cited in Lennie Kronisch, "Elisabeth Kübler-Ross: Messenger of Love," *Yoga Journal* 11 (November–December 1976): 19.

7. Kathryn Hulme, *The Nun's Story* (Boston: Little, Brown and Co., 1956), 14–15.

Chapter 4

From Survivors to Pioneers

Ralph Braun was a true pioneer. He was born on December 18, 1940, and raised in Winamac, Indiana. When he was six years old, he was diagnosed with muscular dystrophy, a disease marked by a gradual wasting and weakening of skeletal muscles. The doctors told his parents he would not live to be a teenager. They were wrong. Necessity is the mother of invention, and Ralph's physical limitations fueled his determination to live as independently as possible. He was a hard worker. At the age of fourteen, he started using a wheelchair. At fifteen, he and his father created a motorized wagon to help him get around. Five years later, he developed a motorized scooter called the tri-wheeler using parts from his cousin's farm. The tri-wheeler helped him to conserve energy and to commute to his job as a quality control manager at a nearby manufacturer. When the company moved several miles away, he equipped an old mail carrier jeep with a hydraulic tailgate lift and hand controls to accommodate his tri-wheeler. It was the first known wheelchair lift.

Assembling tri-wheelers became a full-time job for Braun. He gathered a team to help with his work and turned his parent's garage into a workplace that evolved into BraunAbility. It was incorporated in 1972 and became a leading manufacturer of wheelchair lifts and ramps for paratransit vans and cutaway buses. It produced wheelchair-accessible minivans, wheelchair platform lifts, and personal-use products. What set BraunAbility apart from other mobility product manufacturers was Ralph's focus on providing mobility solutions that met the individual needs of each customer. He had a network of dealers across the country that evaluated individuals according to their needs, circumstances, and level of disability. Braun and his son Todd were owners of the NASCAR team, Braun Racing. President Barack Obama named him a "champion of change" in honor of his dedication to improving the lives of people with physical disabilities. Just a week before he died, Ralph was honored with the Support of the Guard and Reserves Patrol Award for his support of his employees who serve in the military.

Ralph was married, had five children, and was an inventor, entrepreneur, and CEO. His adversities in life were met with innovation, adaptive skills, and hard work. Ralph died on February 8, 2013, in Winamac. His five life lessons were "put the customer first," "no excuses," "surround yourself with good people," "never stop improving," and "believe in your God-given ability."[1]

What Next?

After the rather intense diagnostic tests and initial treatment plan during the acute stage of a serious disease are over, it is common to experience new anxieties and uncertainties at the beginning of maintenance treatment. Life is different, but it settles into routine again. We may miss the special attention from family and friends that once animated our days during initial treatment, and the steady stream of flowers, food, gifts, and wishes also diminishes. Beginning life after the dust settles can be anticlimactic. We may feel let down because the critical stage with its support from health care professionals has passed. We may feel void, at loose ends, or even abandoned. If a large part of our self-identity was being a patient, that has been greatly diminished. We pause and reflect. Life will not return to what it was. How has my disease changed me? What new revelations did chronic health concerns awaken in me?

How chronic disease changes our lives depends on us. Inner strengths and new gifts are positive discoveries and can be shared with others who have chronic diseases. Grievances, petty annoyances, and resentments that were present before the disease, but suspended during the high stress of diagnosis and treatment, may resurface. We, and others, might return to irritating pre-disease patterns or resume old arguments and conflicts. Conversely, if we look on the bright side, these negative circumstances may simply disappear in the sunlight of the present because we are so grateful for the gift of life. Many disagreeable things are no longer a burden because life has a new sweetness. Having a long-term disease may teach us the importance of cultivating a practice of gratitude, which produces a greater appreciation of all that is beautiful.

Shakespeare wrote, "Whereof what's past is prologue."[2] And so it is. We have a chance to begin again. Our life changed because we had a personal encounter with a difficult transition. There is no going back to the good old days. Now we need to move on. We approach our new life and gaze as we stand at its threshold. New life can be a fascinating venture, and we proceed with caution, trepidation, joy, and wondrous anticipation. Our identity as survivors came about through dealing with difficult health care events. Now a new identity presents itself: that of a pioneer.

The possibility of self-discovery and authentic wholeness at this stage of the journey are exemplified by the following proverb: A stream was moving across the countryside, experiencing little difficulty. It ran around rocks and through mountains. Then it arrived at a desert. Just as it had crossed every other barrier, the stream tried to cross this one, but it found that as fast as it ran into the sand, the waters disappeared. After many attempts, it appeared that there was no way it could continue the journey. Then a voice came in the wind, "If you stay the way you are, you cannot cross the sands. To go further, you will have to lose yourself." "But if I lose myself," the stream cried, "I will never know what I am supposed to do." "Oh, on the contrary," said the voice, "if you lose yourself, you will become more than you ever dreamed you could be." So, the stream surrendered to the drying sun. And the clouds into which it was formed were carried by the raging wind for many miles. Once it crossed the desert, the stream poured down from the skies, fresh and clean and full of the energy that comes from storms.

Two Roads Emerge

We step over the threshold and see two paths available to us: one is short, the other long. Which path will we trod? After their acute illness, survivors choose either to roost as settlers or to roam as pioneers. Settlers sink their roots into the dirt of their old ways of life. They see no reason or need for change and slip back into their pre-diagnostic bad habits. They stay in their comfort zones and are complacent and content with what is easy, comfortable, and mediocre. Their lives can resemble hamsters running on the wheels in their cages. They swap grim stories about their ailments and worry about their return. Their interior lives are unusually inert as they go through the motions in their days.

Pioneers' interior lives move ahead. They find opportunities to love and be loved in their days. Their lives can resemble wild horses running on the prairie. Pioneers are adventurers on the journey of life. They take the risks of innovators on the move with new projects or interests. Just think of how many helpful organizations were established by people who had serious diseases. Pioneers thrive on challenges to work, play, live, and pray with fervor. Notes from "My Symphony" by William Henry Channing drift into a pioneer's lifestyle:

> To live content with small means.
> To seek elegance rather than luxury,
>   and refinement rather than fashion.
> To be worthy, not respectable,
>   and wealthy, not rich.
> To study hard, think quietly, talk gently,
>   act frankly, to listen to stars, birds, babes,
>   and sages with open heart, to bear all cheerfully,
>   do all bravely, await occasions, hurry never.
> In a word to let the spiritual,
>   unbidden and unconscious,
>   grow up through the common.
> This is to be my symphony.[3]

Life-defeating choices support a settler orientation. Life-enhancing choices support a pioneer orientation. Being human, we by nature often vacillate in decision-making throughout our lives. Each day we make conscious or unconscious, easy or hard decisions that result in being happy, sad, healthy, sick, creative, or unimaginative. We experience the full continuum, from lighting the candles to cursing the darkness. However, we can endeavor to overcome settler decisions if we try hard to think like pioneers. This is a call to take charge and forge ahead with our new lease on life. During onset treatment, the reins were in the hands of doctors. Maintenance treatments are in our hands. As we know, health challenges can put us to the test, but they can also bring out the best in us.

Moving ahead means improving our physical, mental, and spiritual landscape. If we are frightened about persevering, we need to remember how far we have already come. We have trekked over high mountains and through deep valleys we never knew existed. And that which is behind us gives us the push we need to travel on the road ahead of us. Through the physical, mental, and spiritual difficulties we experienced on the uneven road of fragile health, new life was born that will sustain us on the pioneer road, where we learn to keep our thoughts on sunrises rather than sunsets. Ralph Braun advises us: "I was frustrated then—and sometimes now I am, too—because of certain things I couldn't do for myself. I'd rather I didn't need help going to the restroom, taking a shower, or eating. … But I have learned to handle those frustrations and deal with them because that's the way it is. I know I have more to offer to society than just sitting around and worrying about a few frustrations and my own discomfort. To do otherwise seems self-indulgent and wrong."[4]

If we choose to be a pioneer, it might be a good idea to take along a walking stick as a reminder that we need physical, mental, and spiritual support on our new journey. The walking stick is also a reminder that being healthy does not require perfect physical, mental, or spiritual well-being. If we remain calm and objective and treat ourselves with compassion and tolerance during difficulties, it can provide an affirmation of our humanity and can be a source of personal growth.

Have Courage to Embrace Constructive Change

The fundamental characteristic of a pioneer is the courage to take the first step toward life-enhancing behavior. The difficulties that are born of chronic disease may be seen as compost, unpleasant and not valuable in itself. However, when used well, compost produces verdant growth. The negative plateaus we experience with chronic disease can be seen as bleak encounters with winter. They are times of low energy and poor function. Thoughts may be muted, minds muddled, and actions slowed. Nevertheless, life without obstacles leads nowhere, and negative plateaus can be compared to time within a compost pile. Like a garden under winter's snow, we wait for the growth of spring.

Courage is essential to change our self-defeating ways to life-giving ones. It is tough to break a bad habit, but since we have been through the complexities and long-term effects of our disease, the odds are in our favor. However, we cannot just stop bad habits. We need internal fortitude—this is the first step—then we can find support from organizations, people, and other sound sources. Another major help is to identify and integrate a good habit to replace a bad habit. Instead of impulsive eating, we can say the rosary—its mysteries can give us plenty of spiritual nourishment. Instead of throwing things when we are angry, we utilize a punching bag. If we are down in the dumps and can only see a blank wall in front of us, we can put bright and uplifting banners on it. If the wall is black, we can paint on stars, comets, meteors, and galaxies. When we are feeling out of sorts, we can write down ten good things about ourselves, pause, and say, "That's right!" We hold on to our dreams with faith and strive to make them real. Courage and determination help us to do things that are creative and unique.

Recognize When You Can't Go It Alone

Once upon a time, a little girl was lost in a large wheat field. Her parents called in the neighbors to help find her, but all was in vain. Although they shouted and searched, they could not find the little girl. Finally, on the third day, the father said to the townspeople, "Let us all join hands and go through the field in a line." No one said, "I must tend to my crops" or "I have too many things to do." They immediately stopped whatever they were doing to pursue a common purpose and greater good. In no time, the child was found

Sometimes we must let go of what we think is best, pull together, and find a good solution to a difficult problem. If we meet people who know more than we do, we keep our eyes and ears open, for learning is a lifelong experience. The world is varied beyond our expectations and there are always opportunities to learn and teach. Serious problems demand that we anchor our feet firmly on the ground. From that stance, we can see more easily how we are interdependent on each other: "God's dream is that you and I and all of us will realize that we are family, that we are made for togetherness, for goodness, and for compassion."[5] The goodness of others can come from a horrifying situation, and solving that situation can be the cause of great joy.

For Christians, the epitome of working together is making room for God and letting ourselves be loved by him. During the duration of our disease, we may see how the various finite satisfactions we seek are fleeting and how we ache for the infinite. Finite satisfactions are good, but we are deceiving ourselves if we expect too much from them. They are pleasant in their time and place but cannot quench our longing for something more. When we realize finite goods do not fully satisfy us, we know that more of the same is only a delusion. There are many of us who live within the trends of today but when life turns us around, we realize there is much more to life than what is currently fashionable. We have learned that craving for superficial negative things may be an unknown camouflage for a deep spiritual thirst or an unidentified spiritual void.

Today, God is often relegated to the background, but he is the foundation of our equilibrium, and his rightful place is on the front lines of our lives. If we want to live a wholesome life, we need to make room for God. To support this, it would be beneficial to have reminders of him, or holy people we associate with him, in our living spaces. These could be statues or pictures, holy books or cards, inspirational quotes or other visual aids that lead our thoughts to God and remind us that his grace is working in our days. Recognizing God's love for us awakens our hearts to his divine light. Elizabeth of the Trinity reminds us that our challenge is to let ourselves be loved by God. To be still and quiet in a peaceful setting for five minutes two times a day, while relaxing in God's love without saying a word, is a very peaceful prayer. God loves us more than we can possibly realize. To ease into a cozy chair and let his love gently saturate us like a warm healing balm can revive our tired mind and drooping spirit. Because we are receptive to God loving us, we are able to love ourselves more.

Be a Beam of Light for Others to Follow

Once we have habituated courage and accepted others' love, we can in turn become beacons and guides to others, who are starting their journeys as pioneers. Love is the foundation of all virtues, or good habits of the heart. If we strive to embrace these virtues, then we learn to value people for who they are rather than for their usefulness. We realize that individual achievement is not pursued at the expense of justice or of community. If a fellow human being is worried or unhappy, it should be noticed and addressed with love: "Let love be genuine. Abhor what is evil; hold fast to what is good. Love one another with brotherly affection. Outdo one another in showing honor" (Rom. 12:9–10, ASV).

Love is a gift of self. Teresa of Calcutta wrote, "Give love to your children, your wife or husband, to a next door neighbor. . . . Let no one ever come to you without leaving better or happier. Be the living expression of God's kindness; kindness in your face, kindness in your eyes, kindness in your smile, kindness in your warm greeting."[6] Indeed, these are sure steps to well-being. Love takes us beyond ourselves. It is a decisive action for another that often takes the place of something we want to do for ourselves. A healthy physical, mental, and spiritual orientation is love-giving and life-enhancing. This can be more prominent when our physical health is not first-rate. In fact, a person with physical limitations can be more wholesome than a person with perfect physical health. Our conduct reveals more about who we are than our appearance or what we do. Maintaining order with a positive attitude, sense of humor, and trustworthiness discloses more about us than our performance of a task. The love we put into a work of service is of greater importance than the status of that service.

If we look in the mirror and smile then pass that smile on to others, it may make their day. If we take time to praise others and show an interest and enthusiasm about their projects, they will feel affirmed. Kindness propels us to love people even when they disagree or disappoint us, and not to doubt the love others have for us. A Japanese proverb says, "One kind word can warm three winter months." Isn't that true?

Oremus, Let Us Pray

Finally, pioneers cannot achieve or maintain their forward momentum without prayer. Prayer is wonderfully varied: Adoration, silently beholding Jesus face to face through faith, is a most beautiful form of worship. Intercessory prayer for others bonds them with God even though they may be unaware of it. Praising God lifts our hearts in good times and bad. Sometimes a prayer can be a quiet sigh or a painful cry.

And there are prayers of contrition that express our sorrow for having offended God and hurt others. We can meditate on stories in the gospels. Deep prayer is silent, loving attentiveness to God. Whatever the style, our prayers flow through the days like gentle streams linking us to heaven and bringing us closer to God and to our authentic selves. Prayer can be miraculous as it guides people to God's truth, and somehow their eyes of greed and power change to eyes of love and mercy.

Prayer as a long-term commitment has its challenges. In time it becomes a blessed routine, independent of feelings that are accidental to the primary purpose of prayer, which is communion with God in faith. It sustains and nourishes our spiritual life. The water from God's wellspring of wisdom is the only thing that can quench our deepest thirst. Jesus is our best teacher. He reveals God's love to us. He is the most splendid evidence that God exists. Prayer infuses love into our day and sustains perseverance and hope in our lives. Prayer is our language of faith. John of the Cross wrote: "Faith lies beyond all this understanding, taste, feeling, and imagining ... However impressive may be one's knowledge or experience of God, that knowledge or experience will have no resemblance to God and amount to very little. ... Those who want to reach union with God should advance neither by understanding, nor by the support of their own experience, nor by feeling or imagination, but by belief in God's being."[7]

God is the source and substance of reality. He is omniscient and omnipotent, yet he works through us. God is like a circle whose center is everywhere and whose circumference is nowhere. He is infinite and omnipresent yet dwells in the center of our hearts. God is very near, yet his nearness remains veiled in exquisite mystery. We only grasp at straws to describe him. Yet it is in God that we live and move and have our being, and in whom we seek and serve, each of us reflecting a facet of his image:

> Thou art the source that causes our river to flow.
> Thou art hidden in Thy essence, but seen by Thy
>   bounties.
> Thou art like the water, and we like the millstone.
> Thou art like the wind, and we like the dust;
> The wind is unseen, but the dust is seen by all.
> Thou art the Spring, and we the sweet green garden;
> Spring is not seen, though its gifts are seen.
> Thou art the Soul, we as hand and foot;
> Soul instructs hand and foot to hold and take.
> Thou art as Reason, we like the tongue;
> 'Tis reason that teaches the tongue to speak.
> Thou art as Joy, and we are laughing;
> The laughter is the consequence of the joy.
> Our every motion every moment testifies,
> For it proves the presence of the everlasting God.[8]

Notes

1. "Father of the Mobility Movement—Ralph Braun," accessed August 30, 2022, https://www.braunability.com/us/en/about-us/ralph-braun.html.

2. William Shakespeare, *The Tempest*, ed. Barbara A. Mowat and Paul Werstine (Washington, DC: Folger Shakespeare Library, 2015), 2.1.289.

3. William Henry Channing, "My Symphony," *All Poetry* (blog), accessed August 30, 2022, https://allpoetry.com/poem/8557243-My-Symphony-by-William-Ellery-Channing.

4. Ralph W. Braun, *Rise Above: How One Man's Search for Mobility Helped the World Get Moving* (Winamac, IN: Braun Corporation, 2010), chap. 5, https://www.braunability.com/us/en/about-us/rise-above/chapter-5.html.

5. Desmond Tutu, interviewed in "Desmond Tutus's Recipe for Peace," Beliefnet, April 2004, https://www.beliefnet.com/inspiration/2004/04/desmond-tutus-recipe-for-peace.aspx.

6. Mother Teresa, *100 Inspirational Quotes* (Delhi: Penguin Books India, 2016), 59.

7. John of the Cross, *The Ascent of Mount Carmel*, in *The Collected Works of St. John of the Cross*, trans. Kieran Kavanaugh and Otilio Rodriguez (Washington, DC: ICS Publications, 1991), II.4.2–4.

8. Jalal ad-Din Rumi, "The Gifts of the Beloved," in *The Sacred Books and Early Literature of the East*, vol. 8, *Medieval Persia* (Park Austin, and Lipscomb, 1917; Fordham University, 1998), https://sourcebooks.fordham.edu/source/1250rumi-masnavi.asp.

Chapter 5

The Elders among Us

Tony Snow (1955–2008) was a journalist, political commentator, television news anchor, White House press secretary, and syndicated columnist. What he wrote about his cancer is worth many meditations:

> I don't know why I have cancer, and I don't much care. It is what it is, a plain and indisputable fact. Yet even while staring into a mirror darkly, great and stunning truths began to take shape. Our maladies define a central feature of our existence: We are fallen. We are imperfect. Our bodies give out. But, despite this——or because of it——God offers the possibility of salvation and grace. We don't know how the narrative of our lives will end, but we get to choose how to use the interval between now and the moment we meet our Creator face-to-face.
>
> Second, we need to get past the anxiety. The mere thought of dying can send adrenaline flooding through your system. A dizzy, unfocused panic seizes you. Your heart thumps; your head swims. You think of nothingness and swoon. You fear partings; you worry about the impact on family and friends. You fidget and get nowhere. To regain footing, remember that we were

born not into death, but into life—and that the journey continues after we have finished our days on the earth. We accept this on faith, but that faith is nourished by a conviction that stirs even within many non-believing hearts—an intuition that the gift of life, once given, cannot be taken away. Those who have been stricken enjoy the special privilege of being able to fight with their might, main, and faith to live fully, richly, exuberantly—no matter how their days may be numbered.

Third, we can open our eyes and hearts. God relishes surprise. We want lives of simple, editable ease—smooth, even trials as far as the eye can see—but God likes to go off-road. He provokes us with twists and turns. He places us in predicaments that seem to defy our endurance and comprehension—and yet don't. By his love and grace, we persevere. The challenges that make our hearts leap and stomachs churn invariably strengthen our faith and grant measures of wisdom and joy we would not experience otherwise. . . .

The moment you enter the Valley of the Shadow of Death, things change. You discover that Christianity is not something doughy, passive, pious, and soft. Faith may be the substance of things hoped for, the evidence of things not seen. But it also draws you into a world shorn of fearful caution. The life of belief teems with thrills, boldness, danger, shocks, reversals, triumphs, and epiphanies. . . . There's nothing wilder than a life of humble virtue—for it is through selflessness and service that God wrings from our bodies and spirits the most we ever could give, the most we ever could offer, and the most we ever could do.

Finally, we can let love change everything. . . . We get repeated chances to learn that life is not about us, that we acquired purpose and satisfaction by sharing in God's love for others.

Sickness gets us part way there. It reminds us of our limitations and dependence. But it also gives us a chance to serve the healthy.[1]

Tony Snow's excellent interpretation of what it means to have cancer is also applicable to other serious diseases and even to the aging process.

A Journey toward Wisdom

Although people are living longer today than at any other time in history, the number of our years on this earth is unknown to us. Life is rarely predictable, and no one really knows what aging will bring. This is one reason why old age may be the most medically challenging chapter in the book of life: "To know how to grow old is the master work of wisdom, and one of the most difficult chapters in the great art of living."[2] It is true that when experiencing the rigors of serious sickness or dark days in general, nothing may make sense. However, we try to appreciate life's blessings and manage its burdens. Things can begin to calm down, come together to make some reasonable sense, and impart unforeseen wisdom.

When we reach what we think is midlife, we may give this thought some reflection: We hope for a good and long journey on our road of life but know it can come to an end at any time. Focusing on the long road we wonder, What does it mean to age, to be an elder? There are many answers. Perhaps, like beauty, old age is in the eye of the beholder. At age twenty, we may have thought fifty was old. At fifty that number changed to seventy. Or is "old" primarily based on an objective number of years? Numbers are not the real answer.

Courage through Chronic Disease

It is not uncommon to know someone in his or her twenties who acts like a grouchy old person or someone in their eighties who has a delightful disposition and is young at heart.

Alternatively, is "old" more philosophical and determined by how we react to the experiences in life, the so-called good or bad things that come our way? The sharp distinction between the two can diminish as we get along in years, because we can develop a tolerance for and understanding of opposing points of view. This doesn't mean being spineless about where we stand but broadening our perspective by replacing snap judgments with an open-minded interest. For example, the slowing down that comes with aging can give senior folks the time to look for beauty in things not noticed before: The autumn leaves, winter frost, spring flowers, and summer sky take on a deeper meaning. The grandeur of nature may have been unnoticed because of a previously hectic lifestyle. Now it is time to stop and ponder.

This reflection on the meaning of aging may begin a journey into the wisdom within us that we did not know existed. Even in our older years, we strive to become who we are meant to be, and a large part of this is through discovering wisdom. As physical strength and beauty fade, beauty of heart, mind, and soul can grow brighter as the years roll by. Each elder person has a set of values and beliefs that are manifest in who he or she is, affects what he or she does, and shapes his or her interpretation of life. The quality of these attributes, reflected in what we think and expressed in what we say, transmits certain aspects about ourselves to those around us. Socrates said, "There is nothing which for my part I like better, Cephalus, than conversing with aged men; for I regard them as travelers who have gone a journey which I too may have to go, and of whom I ought to enquire, whether the way is smooth and easy, or rugged and difficult."[3] If we think about it, we have many pearls of wisdom to give to others. If we grow through the storms of aging, we will have even more pearls to give.

Aging can enlighten us and those around us. Many years bring insights that are gleaned from knowing more about history, personal struggle, obstacles faced, losses endured, milestones celebrated, and risks taken. With the passage of time, the high emotions of youth can diminish and be replaced with a soothing composure. The testimony of an older person can give hope to the younger person who is experiencing a traumatic or life-changing event. Elders show young people who are experiencing troubles that their world has not crumbled. Consider the following fable:

An old man whom villagers trusted and revered was often sought out for his wisdom. A farmer came to him and said, "Wise man, I need your help. A terrible thing has happened. My old horse died, and I have no animal to help me plow my field. Is this not the worst thing that could possibly happen?" The old man said, "Maybe so, maybe not." The farmer got a younger horse and could not wait to tell the old man, "Isn't this the best thing that ever happened?" The wise man said, "Maybe so, maybe not." The lively young horse threw the farmer's son, causing him to break his leg. "Isn't this the worst thing that could happen to my son?" the farmer told the man. "Maybe so, maybe not," the wise man replied. The next day soldiers came and conscripted every young man, except the farmer's son, for the army.

From Regret to Personal Development

When we look back on our lives, we may experience regret, especially for the "I should haves." We may regret not being kinder to our siblings, listening to our parents, or spending enough time with our families; not getting that degree or job; or not making that move or taking that trip. If we brood over these past events and merge them with other disappointments, unfinished projects, mistakes, or other negative occurrences, they can lead to discouraging thought patterns that drain energy and limit creative thinking that are necessary for the present. The memory of what we did not do then should not darken the light of what we can do now. We must strive to avoid the pitfalls of negative ruminations.

Another pitfall is to compare the quality of our life with that of our younger selves, a friend, a family member, or an acquaintance. No two people are exactly alike, and thank goodness for that. Healthy aging is becoming comfortable with who we are in our uniqueness, with no regret about who we are not or wish that we were like someone else. As we get older, we can also experience regret over a gradual loss of vision, hearing, energy, or memory. Loss of family and friends through distance or death is more common than at any other stage of life. However, to view aging as a continuing series of losses only leads to a downward spiral. As we descend, we lose sight of opportunities for greater maturity.

The positive side of regret is to look at the evil things we have done to ourselves and others in the past and to be contrite for them now. Certain vices, such as pride and greed, blind us to the good around and within us because we are so engrossed in ourselves. We have made great strides forward if we are now genuinely sorry for the times we were abusive, ruined someone's reputation, habitually lied, stole, cheated, or participated in other vices. Our sorrow includes a sincere promise not to participate in evil activities again. Forgiveness for these actions is an ongoing necessity if we want inner peace. The poet Frederick Tennyson wrote,

> Two aged men, that had been foes for life,
>   Met by grave and wept—and in those tears
>   They wash'd away the memory of their strife;
> Then wept again the loss of all those years.[4]

Can we improve our personality at this late date? The invitation to be a better person is always before us. In particular, contentment, the opposite of regret, is accessible as we get on in years: stubborn teenagers can mellow as adults. Hard-driving adults can become gentle elders. Elder years give us the freedom not to worry about making the grade or getting ahead. We learn to settle in and be content with what we have. We can go from schedules and deadlines to quiet and ease, from accessories to essence, from running around to reflective walking, from fast food to leisurely dining. Indeed, a blessing of the elder years is experiencing the multifaceted beauty of simplicity.

Likewise, accepting age-associated losses is a sound addition to our repertoire of wisdom. Being patient as we adjust to each loss, and accepting that this is part of aging, may bring much more to light. A weakness in old age can prompt a new strength like greater sensitivity to the needs of others. More effort to do simple things can evolve into greater patience with ourselves. If we use a cane or walker, we can experience an unspoken bond with others who use walking aids. Decreased muscle strength can result in a greater companionship with those we call when we need assistance. The loss of a driver's license can turn drivers into friends. We know the value of waiting and trying again. We may do physical tasks differently, and they may turn out better than before.

We may not have the agility to plant seeds in the fields, but we can plant them in the hearts or in the souls of others. It is uplifting to find new and positive aspects of ourselves, of others, and of God after a loss. The spiritual realm has many aspects on which to ruminate, and one can make great strides in spiritual growth during the elder years. As a person experiences physical loss, there can be spiritual gain. Prayer energizes spiritual development and brings us nearer to God.

Another way to improve our personality is to increase our knowledge about subjects that we did not recognize or fully appreciate before. One outdated myth is that elders are useless. We are never too old to create something new. Psalm 92:14 tells us, "They shall still bring forth fruit in old age; they shall be full of sap and green" (RSV). Elders are useless only if they choose to be useless. An Irish proverb tells us: "The older the fiddle the sweeter the tune." We may be old, but we need not think old or feel old in our heart. In other cultures, silver hair and wrinkles are signs of wisdom and service. Let us "bring it on" here. How often have we noticed that some silver-haired people can speak more by their being than by their words? Each elder person has his or her own interpretation of beauty. Perhaps creating something beautiful will neutralize the negative stereotypes of aging. Seniors who play a musical instrument, or who can otherwise entertain people, can perform at an assisted-living facility or direct a talent show. They can volunteer in parish activities or tend a garden. They can make phone calls for a good cause, start a monthly book club or weekly singing group, launch a petition, write an editorial, call a congressperson, or volunteer at a community service project. Other options are starting or participating in a club or prayer group, tutor at a grammar school, teach an adult to read, or read to children or adults.

This opportunity is not lost even if we are uprooted from a familiar routine or a dear home we enjoyed for decades and relocated to a senior apartment or an institution for elder care. After a period of adjustment to a new environment, do we choose to sit inside and vegetate or get out and explore?

Grace at the End of Life

Dying is a fact. What should we do when medicine cannot save our life? A long tradition prevailed from the time of Hippocrates until the middle of the twentieth century. It was the physician who said what should be done in the face of devastating disease. Today, what the patient wants is taken under consideration. This can still be guided by the principles of Hippocratic medicine: "To do away with the sufferings of the sick, to lessen the violence of their diseases, and to refuse to treat those who are overmastered by their diseases."[5]

Human life can be seen as a gift from God given to us for a certain amount of time. The *Baltimore Catechism* tells us that God made us "to know Him, to love Him, and to serve Him in this world, and to be happy with Him forever in heaven."[6] We are given the gift of life in order to learn how to love the Creator of life through appreciating and caring for his creation. If we have a serious illness, we know in a deeper way how each moment of life is precious. We extend this thought to the last moments in life because we are still a part of life. However, this does not mean preserving life at all costs or ending it when it seems burdensome or useless.

A sound moral guide is found in Pope Pius XII's Allocution to the International Congress of Anesthesiologists, given on November 24, 1957. He stated that we are normally obliged to use only ordinary means to preserve life. Ordinary means are those things we are obliged to do. Extraordinary means are those things we may do but are not obliged to do, because the treatment would be too costly, too burdensome, or too painful, or because the procedure would not offer a reasonable expectation of benefit. Does common sense support a patient's remaining on artificial respiration, nutrition, and hydration when body systems are shutting down and death is imminent? It is important to protect, until the moment of natural death, the dignity of the person. A balanced perspective aided by prayer helps us with solutions for end-of-life issues. We need not deplete all our energy or use every possible resource to cling to life when medical treatment is no longer effective. Relief from pain and distress should be provided even if we can foresee but do not intend the possible shortening of life. Palliative care and hospice, along with careful pain management and sound support systems, can lighten the burdens of the dying process. This may even be the impetus for spiritual growth by strengthening faith and increasing awareness of God's presence. As we work through and respect the dying process, we may receive unanticipated graces. Even if our life is nearing its end, we can still be good stewards of life. Caring for people near the end of life should include the concept of healing, which involves arriving at a peaceful place before the time of death.

Elders among Us

Assisted suicide and euthanasia are becoming more popular. We must be constantly vigilant against this current trend, which is a conscious and erroneous ideology that taking one's life is freedom of choice and euthanasia is death with dignity. Our dignity is based not on what we can do or how we look but on the fact that we are children of God. We affirm the dignity of life by practical, quality palliative services. We may sit at the bedside of someone who is dying. There is nothing we can do to prevent dying; however, a simple prayer can be comforting and reassuring. Perhaps quiet prayers and a loving presence are just what the person needs. A healing presence may bring forth in the one who is dying an inner resource to see beyond present limitations. When people express a wish to die, it may be interpreted as a need to know if they are still loved, special, and worthwhile. Perhaps they want to know they will not be abandoned or seen as a burden. Perhaps they want reassurance that they will grow in and through their disease. It may be a plea that they will be cared for even though they are not the same as they were before. People who verbalize a plea to die may not be able to verbalize a cry to live.

Perhaps our greatest resource in old age is prayer. With the lessons in faith to guide us and God's grace to strengthen us, old age can be very fruitful. Faith in God keeps us moving ahead and helps us draw on our inner reserves of strength during difficult days. Faith guides us to be gracious and understanding as the infirmities of old age come our way. Upon reflection, we have a deeper understanding of our past successes, a general satisfaction and appreciation about the life we have lived, and a respect for the spiritual dimension. The definition of prayer broadens to include spending quiet time in the company of Jesus or resting in the presence of God.

A man's daughter asked the local priest to come and pray with her father. When the priest arrived, he found the man lying in bed with his head propped up on the pillows. An empty chair sat beside his bed. The priest assumed that the old fellow had been informed of his visit. "I guess you were expecting me," he said. "No, who are you?" said the father. The priest told him his name and then remarked, "I saw the empty chair and I thought you knew I was going to show up." "Oh yes, the chair," said the bedridden man, "Would you mind closing the door?" Puzzled, the priest shut the door. "I have never told anyone this, not even my daughter," said the man. "But all of my life I have never known how to really pray. At church I used to hear the priest talk about prayer, but it went right over my head. I abandoned any serious attempt at prayer until one day, four years ago, my best friend said to me 'Johnny, prayer is just a simple matter of having a conversation with Jesus. Here is what I suggest. Sit down in a chair; place an empty chair in front of you, and in faith see Jesus on the chair. It's not spooky because he promised, *I will be with you always.* Then just speak to him in the same way you are doing with me right now.' So, I tried it, and I've liked it so much that I do it a couple of hours every day. I am careful though. If my daughter saw me talking to an empty chair, she would either have a nervous breakdown or send me off to the funny farm." The priest was deeply moved by the story and encouraged the old man to continue on the journey. Then he anointed him and returned to the church.

Elders among Us

Two nights later, the daughter called to tell the priest that her father had died that afternoon. "Did he die in peace?" he asked. "Yes, when I left the house at about two o'clock, he called me over to his bedside, told me he loved me and kissed me on the cheek. When I got back from the store an hour later, I found him dead. But there was something strange about his death. Apparently, just before Daddy died, he leaned over and rested his head on the chair beside the bed. What do you make of that?"

There is more to death that can be grasped in human terms. We have neither the vocabulary nor the knowledge to adequately understand what happens after death. As humans it is beyond us. God's unconditional love never fails for those who hope in him, and its mystery is the wellspring of true joy, which leads to serenity of soul and a peaceful death. Julian of Norwich wrote, "There is no creature that is made that may (fully) know how much and how sweetly and how tenderly our Maker loveth us. And therefore we may with grace and His help stand in spiritual beholding, with everlasting marvel of this high, overpassing, inestimable Love that Almighty God hath to us of His Goodness."[7]

> We seem to give them back to you, O God, who gave them to us. Yet as you did not lose them in giving, so we do not lose them by their return. . . . Life is eternal and love immortal, and death is only an horizon, and an horizon is nothing save the limit of our sight. Lift us up, strong Son of God, that we may see further; cleanse our eyes that we may see more clearly; draw us closer to yourself that we may know ourselves to be nearer to our loved ones who are with you.[8]

Notes

1. Tony Snow, "Cancer's Unexpected Blessings," *Christianity Today*, July 20, 2007, reprinted in "Tony Snow's Testimony," *Poetic Expressions* (blog), accessed September 20, 2022, https://www.poeticexpressions.co.uk/t-snow/.

2. Henri Frédéric Ameil, *Amiel's Journal*, trans. Humphrey Ward (MacMillan, 1889; Project Gutenberg, 2016), https://www.gutenberg.org/files/8545/8545-h/8545-h.htm#link2H_PREF.

3. Plato, *The Republic*, trans. Benjamin Jowett, in *Plato, Great Books of the Western World* (Chicago: Encyclopaedia Britannica, 1990), I.328.

4. Frederick Tennyson, "The Golden City," in *The Shorter Poems of Frederick Tennyson*, ed. Charles Tennyson (London: MacMillan, 1913), 150.

5. Hippocrates, *The Art*, in Hippocrates, vol. 2, ed. T.E. Page et al., trans. W.H.S. Jones, *Loeb Classical Library* (Cambridge, MA: Harvard University Press, 1923), 193.

6. Bennet Kelley, *Saint Joseph Baltimore Catechism*, rev. ed. no. 2 (New York: Catholic Book Publishing, 1969), 9.

7. Julian of Norwich, *Revelations of Divine Love*, ed. Grace Warrack (Methuen, 1901; Project Gutenberg, 2016), chap. 6, https://www.gutenberg.org/files/52958/52958-h/52958-h.htm.

8. This prayer, attributed to Bede Jarrett, was published in *The Catholic Prayer Book from Downside Abbey*, ed. David Foster (Edinburgh: T&T Clark, 1999), 130.

Chapter 6

The Emperor and the Children

A most dreaded and feared disease that has been with us for over five thousand years is cancer. Dr. Siddhartha Mukherjee's title for his Pulitzer Prize winning book is *The Emperor of All Maladies*. That is what cancer is. Cancer is a general title that includes a complex collection of disorders people get for reasons whose causes are not completely clear. No age is free from cancer, but it is most devastating when it is diagnosed in children. No one can adequately describe the shock. Like a vicious storm, with deep heart-rending turbulences, it invades the family. Initially, it feels like a tidal wave, followed by an ongoing ebb and flow of hopes, disappointments, emotional ups and downs, and unimaginable turmoil.

During the routine days of treatments, and tests for treatment effectiveness, unexpected fog can obstruct sensible thinking and leave the child's dear ones in a slump. Parents cannot see what lies ahead and feel lost or disoriented. During these times, it is natural for them to cry until they can cry no more because this is their beloved child. Conflicting periods of interior dark, light, storms, and calm are normal. The interior weather can change due to a specific reason or no apparent reason. Unexpectedly, the fog lifts, the storm calms, and the light shines making it possible to pick up and soldier on.

Dark times are easier to bear when they rest in hope. French writer, Albert Camus, wrote, "O light! This is the cry of all the characters of ancient drama brought face to face with their fate. This last resort was ours, too, and I knew it now. In the middle of winter, I at last discovered that there was in me an invincible summer."[1] Hope is like a shield against despair, struggles, and seemingly dead ends. When all seems dark, hope is the tiny spark of light that helps create conditions conducive to life.

A New Routine

No one can adequately prepare for the responsibility of caring for a child with cancer. There will be sleepless nights, harrowing days, and unexpected trips to the doctor, hospital or emergency room. Adjustments to new people, places, protocols, difficult decisions, and grueling challenges seem endless. However, there is always a brighter side, such as unexpected moments of joy and surges of courage; meeting special people who are generous and loving; encountering wise elders who know the benefits of avoiding negative and despairing thoughts and holding on to what is possible and positive. Indeed, we find stronger endurance in severe struggles, and a deeper appreciation of good things.

For children, experiencing long and difficult cancer treatment can be worse than having the disease. There may be unexpected side effects. Dreaded anticipation or experience of invasive procedures can make the child feel afraid and helpless. Children may struggle to vocalize or understand their fears, and manifest them in depression, sadness, or anger.

But fears may be reduced or revealed through writing, drawing, physical tasks, or other creative activities. Art and music therapists, and recreational and occupational therapists can help in this area. Children may begin to feel more confidence when they have choices available through imaginative modalities, which give them some sense of control in the unfamiliar territories of cancer.

A child's attitude toward his cancer is important. Billy was eleven years old when he was diagnosed with cancer. At that time, he thought that God made each one of us for a different reason. If God gave us a great voice, maybe he wanted us to sing. If God made us seven feet tall, maybe he wanted us to play basketball. When his six-year-old friend Beth died from cancer, he asked his mom, why did God make her born at all? His mom told him that even though she was only six, she changed people's lives. That meant her brother or sister might become a scientist who would help to discover a cure for cancer, because they saw how Beth suffered.

Billy used to wonder why God picked on him and gave him cancer. Maybe it was because he wanted him to become a doctor who takes care of kids with cancer. So, when his little patients would tell him they get so scared, or that he doesn't know how weird it is to be the only bald kid in school, he could tell them, yes, he did because when he was young, he had cancer, was bald, and look at all his hair now.

Mary's greatest pleasure as a child came from sand. Building sandcastles was her delight. Her castle provided a home for a beautiful princess. The walls protected this princess from the crashing ocean waves. Mary dug a trench that surrounded the castle and marveled at the water swirling in her moat. Inevitably, the ocean spilled into the gateway and washed away the castle. Mary didn't fret. She knew she could rebuild the castle. Then, as an older teenager, Mary was diagnosed with cancer. She carried her childhood philosophy into her cancer years. When something became problematic, or no longer worked, she tried something else. She learned how to compensate, found good things in the swirling waters of cancer treatment, and lived courageously with the fluctuations of her disease.

To Be a Child

A child with cancer is still a child. Cancer does not define the child or the parents. People close to the child should try not to describe her by their opinions or concerns about cancer. This emphasizes the disease rather than the child. A child's heart is tender and vulnerable, and it could be harmed by too much cancer talk.

No one knows how a child contracts cancer. A child must understand that her cancer is not her fault, not caused by something she did or did not do, and that no one will catch her cancer. A young child cannot always process what is happening and requires guidance and wisdom from parents and other caring people. Teaching a child about her cancer requires a delicate balance. Both giving too much information and hiding the facts should be avoided. If the information is too limited, the child can imagine that things are worse than they are. Conversely, children can stop listening or just tune out when too much information is dispensed or if there is excessive talk about negative prospects.

It is a good habit for parents to write cancer concerns down as they happen as a defense against forgetting something. If they research these concerns, or are gathering information about cancer, it should be done in moderation. A desperate search for as much data as possible on the internet may lead to erroneous information, or overload resulting in confusion or heightened anxiety. Parents can lose their grip on reality by spending too much time, or placing too much importance on, cancer data from the internet, cancer chat rooms, support groups, or media advertisements.

It is best that cancer news comes from parents. Age-appropriate information can be delivered in a gentle and soft-spoken manner. Addressing the child's medical condition directly, with empathy and clarity, and avoiding platitudes, is the best way to move forward. The child's cancer can be explained with a focus on how the doctors, nurses, and other people will work together to provide the best possible treatment and care. Words used must make the child feel like she is very much the loved child rather than the cancer kid.

During the time Amy's granddaughter, Abigail, was undergoing treatment for leukemia, Amy and Abigail went to the zoo. That was their all-time favorite place. Abigail's hair was beginning to grow back. A little boy came up to her and asked why her hair was so short. She stood up straight, looked him in the eye, and in a very loud voice she said, "Well, I've got cancer!" Although the little boy's mother appeared to be embarrassed, Abigail just went on her way as if nothing happened.

Parents can affirm support by repeating, "We are in this together." Ask the child to repeat what was said to avoid confusion or misunderstanding. Affirm what the child said and give praise when it is correct or adjustments if it is incorrect. Children can pick up big cancer words but they rarely know what they mean. To ask open-ended questions like "What would you like to know?" or "Is there anything you are worried about?" can calm their minds. Parents may be surprised by the aspects of cancer that are most difficult for a child. Not being able to do the things she used to may be more traumatic than her uncertainty about survival. Fears about separation from family can override the fear of death.

Concentrating on the good things of today is living in the present. Each small accomplishment can be an occasion for joy and wonder. Watching ladybugs, making paper airplanes, frosting a cake, or finding a pretty shell on the beach each have their own delight. Dwelling on the good is reassuring. Examples of promoting these little joys include the office manager who set up a jigsaw puzzle in the radiation waiting area and gave parking stickers to her patients, a parent who shared useful financial information, a technician whose warm smile was so reassuring, a nurse who said something funny and made her anxious patients laugh. These are small gifts that beckon a grateful state of mind. We can learn from parents who have traveled this road before us so that parents who travel this road after us may learn from us.

Someone once said that children with cancer are like candles in the wind who accept the possibility that they are in danger of being extinguished by a gust from nowhere, and yet, as they flicker and dance to remain alive, their brilliance challenges the darkness and dazzles those of us who watch their light.

Children with cancer, or any serious disease, may long to feel needed. Mom can help her daughter with cancer feel needed by giving her small jobs to do around the house, like folding clothes, setting the table, or putting things away, while being aware of the child's energy level and attention span. This is giving attention to the child, not to her cancer. Having something to look forward to is very important to a child especially if it is in line with her natural talents or whatever she was interested in before cancer came along.

As cancer progresses, a child's world becomes smaller. The carefree running and playing of yesterday is replaced by being confined to a bed in a room. Their once boundless energy is replaced by fatigue. For older children, an orientation change may take place. Thoughts of the past or plans for the future may merge into the immediacy of today. The child may not want to see friends or pursue her favorite entertainments because she has lost this desire or is just plain tired. Treatments may have worn out a child. Fatigue may cause a child of any age to sleep a lot. How reassuring it is for the child to briefly awaken and find Mom sitting next to her. The child peacefully closes her eyes, she thinks all is well, Mom is here. Mom need not say a word. Her presence says it all.

Focus on the Family

It is an ordinary reaction for parents, and others who love the child, to feel guilt and sadness when that child is diagnosed with cancer. Anger is also common. At diagnosis, anger may be felt toward a spouse, medical personnel, the world, God, or, at times, toward the child. These feelings are normal. The capacity to feel different emotions is part of what makes us human. Fortunately, there is support staff, such as social workers, nurse practitioners, chaplains, child life specialists, and therapists who specialize in cancer, who can help in the care of children and their families.

Cancer changes family dynamics. Family members retain their roles but personality traits may become more intense. Coping with cancer preys on individual weaknesses, causing tempers to flare or be unnaturally suppressed. For those who are closest to the child, it is important to adopt constructive coping mechanisms. They should not smother or hover over the sick child. Neither should they be overly objective and therefore distance themselves from what is taking place. And again, they should not be overly permissive and cater to the child's whims, for example, allowing her to stay up late or have extra snacks.

Siblings are unique individuals who possess their own personalities, needs, and talents, and they will react to cancer differently. They are sons or daughters just as much as the child with cancer. They need respect because of who they are as individuals, not because they are sisters or brothers of the child with cancer. They have their own place in the family unit. How do they feel about their sibling with cancer receiving more attention? What is the sibling really thinking? One sibling may spend lots of time with the child with cancer and another may not. There are many reasons for this. Parents, or others, can make gentle inquiries, while respecting each child's own method of coping.

The oldest child should not be put in an adult role. Older siblings, or siblings who say yes to whatever is asked, should not have responsibilities beyond their capabilities. It is important to reserve some one-on-one time for siblings, so they know they are still important. If they are receptive, help them to discover according to their age and abilities the ways they can be involved in caring for their brother or sister.

The Emperor and the Children

Siblings may not have the words to express their fears, but their body language, such as avoiding eye contact or suddenly refraining from hugs, may show their fear of cancer. To understand their feelings, try to observe the nuances of their behavior, especially if they have never experienced serious illness or the death of a loved one or a pet. They need reassurance that they, or their bad thoughts, didn't cause the cancer. They need to vent their negative feelings, or ask questions about cancer, perhaps to a neutral third party. Parents and other caregivers should watch for signs of jealousy, loneliness, fear, or other emotions. Negative feelings may be eased by running around the backyard, playing basketball, or other vigorous activities. It is better to work through negative feelings than to keep them bottled up inside. Siblings should laugh and have fun with a brother or sister who has cancer. Laughter is very important in daily life.

Boundaries and routine help provide the stability siblings need. Whether they know it or not, children thrive with structure and may become scared or confused when their regular schedule is continually disrupted. As much as possible, try to maintain the same family routine as before the child became ill.

In its own time and way, cancer changes lives. Needless pursuits are laid aside and new life lessons are learned. Looking back on written reflections reveals that hard times are survivable and joyful times are dearly treasured. Finding whimsy or lightness in daily activities, and celebrating age-related milestones, are more significant than ever before. Celebrating normal rites of childhood mitigate managing treatments, tests, and other cancer-related activities.

Budded on Earth to Bloom in Heaven

Death is most tragic when it comes to children. Amid this tragedy, we hold onto the hope of the Christian tradition that death is a door that closes on one's earthly life and opens into an abundant eternal life. This hope has great power to transform the sufferings of cancer as seen, for example, in the story of Rita. Rita was sixteen years old. She had been diagnosed with an aggressive form of cancer the previous year. Although she held on to hope, she knew things did not look good.

Rita's family was loving and strong in faith. Rita had four brothers and sisters. She was the middle child. Although she fought with them, she loved them. For as long as she could remember, her family attended Mass together every Sunday. Her parents sent all their children to Catholic schools. Rita appreciated the sacrifices her parents made for her Catholic education. She loved going to school and learning new things.

Her pastor, Father John, often visited Rita. She liked him, especially when he played his electric guitar and sang with a group at the annual parish festival. Rita and her pastor would talk about many things, including her cancer. He was a good listener. She knew God did not give her cancer. Occasionally they would talk about heaven. Father John said Rita would see her beloved grandfather and dear Aunt Rose there, and although she would miss being with her parents, she would be able to watch over them.

This caused Rita to think about the story her teacher told to her class a few years ago. Long ago, somewhere in the eastern United States, there was a knock at the rectory door. The priest answered and saw a young girl in a white First Communion dress and veil. She told him her mother was very sick. He said he would visit her, which he did. The mother lived alone, and after the visit, the priest noticed a photograph of a young girl on her First Communion day. Since she looked like the girl at the rectory door, the priest asked who she was. "She is my daughter," the woman said. "She died a few years after that picture was taken."

When a child dies, guilt is a common feeling in parents and others dear to the child. The question arises, "Could I have done more?" Loved ones did what was reasonable, but there still is that nagging sensation. Medicine has its limits and they wouldn't have wanted their child to undergo painful experimental treatment. They did the best they could with what was available. Losing a child is hard on a marriage, but this storm can be weathered. Hearts need to mend from guilt, blame, sadness, and betrayal. This is usually a long and painful process and never fully resolved. It has been said that at the death of one's child a part of one's heart is cut away, leaving an empty space. Gradually, the pain and grief lessen, but not completely, because the heart is missing someone very dear.

Faith in God is a huge factor in bringing those who love the child out of the depths of mourning. Parents, and other dear ones, hold on to one another and trust in God to heal their deeply wounded hearts. The complete reason for a child's short life is never known until we pass through the gates of heaven. Losing a child takes so much out of us. However, emptiness can foster new growth. In time we may be able to give back, to bear fruit where we were pruned.

We need to hold on to sound spiritual images to remind us of life after death. The Good Shepherd, Jesus with the children, or other stories in the Bible reminds us of heaven. A deceased child may become more beloved as time goes on. Memories that were fleeting, or were quickly replaced with the busyness of those days, return in a more reflective mode. Many good things are remembered. Wouldn't it be beneficial to record or write about them for the grandchildren or others interested in family history?

A young boy named Rickie is buried in a large cemetery. At the tender age of four, he died quite unexpectedly during a routine operation. His headstone depicts the profile of a little boy in overalls kneeling as if planting flowers into the ground. By this picture are the words, "Budded on earth to bloom in heaven." Aren't we all budded on earth to bloom in heaven?

A Childlike Spirituality

As a child's cancer advances, her spiritual world can become deeper. Her prayer can be amazingly simple and direct. Alphonsus Liguori was a priest, bishop, author, and founder of the Redemptorist religious order. He spent the last nineteen years of his life in chronic pain from severe arthritis. It was so bad he could not lift his head from his chest. He encouraged children of all ages to acquire the habit of speaking to God as if they were alone with him. As their dearest and most loving friend, they speak to him with familiarity. With confidence, they tell him their troubles, joys, and fears. In return, he will answer them, not in audible words, but in words they clearly understand in their heart.

It is beautiful to love God because He is God. A young girl returned home. Her aunt asked her, "Where have you been?" "In church" said the girl. "What were you dong in church on such a lovely day?" her aunt gently inquired. "Praying," said the child. "What were you praying for?" the woman said. "Nothing," said the girl, "I was just loving God." And He loves us, more than we could ever love him.

An old legend about John the Evangelist tells us that he lived to a great old age. As he grew older, his words became fewer. Toward the end of his life, he was content to say to his followers: "Little children, love one another." Someone asked him why he kept repeating the same thing. John replied: "Because that is enough."

A childlike faith is a great grace. Children have a natural ability to pray with simplicity. Their words are honest and plain. Therese of Lisieux's prayer was to the point. She told God what she wanted, quite simply, without splendid phrases or words. She assures us that somehow he always managed to understand her. She was a French Discalced Carmelite nun who died at the age of twenty-four, after suffering from the intense agony of pulmonary tuberculosis for eighteen months. She gave us the precious gift of her "Little Way" that teaches us to love God without pretense, and to serve him with simplicity. The "Little Way" is not related to our age, but to our disposition of the heart. Because God loves us as a good father loves his children, we must respond as children to his love. Therese's daily life was transparently straightforward as she lovingly tended to her duties no matter how insignificant they were. She truly believed the words of Matt. 18:3, "Truly, I say to you, unless you turn and become like children, you will never enter the kingdom of heaven." Therese believed that to be childlike is to remain in the present. If we dwell too much in the past or in the future, we can become discouraged. She helps us to look at whatever happens with the eyes of faith. Wherever she turned, she found God. This was not a sentimental practice, but a learned orientation. She teaches us to try to see holiness wherever we are.

Therese gives us courage to take the next little step. In her autobiography, *Story of a Soul*, she tells us how happy she was to realize she was little, weak, and so imperfect. She remained little before God, which to her meant to recognize her nothingness and expect everything from the good God like a little child expects all things from its father. She counsels us to not be troubled by anything and not to try to make a fortune.

A childlike spiritual orientation keeps a twinkle in our eye, a lightness in our step, wonder in our heart, hope in our soul, and resilience in times of trial. We believe that great trouble can give birth to great good. Yes, at times we have doubts, but when the faith of an innocent child takes over, we can rise above those doubts. Jesus said, "Let the children come to me, and do not hinder them, for to such belongs the kingdom of heaven" (Matt. 19:14). Every child can be seen as a blessing which brings down something of heaven into the midst of our earthly existence. Jesus, the compassionate presence of God the Father, often said, "Do not fear: I am with you" (Isa. 41:10). Childlike spirituality trusts in God and is sung, simply and beautifully, in the hymn, "Jesus Loves Me, This I Know":

When we look with the eyes of a child, we can lose ourselves in wonder, beauty, and the mystery of God. Jesus, the compassionate presence of God the Father, often said, "Do not fear: I am with you" (Isa. 41:10). Childlike spirituality trusts in God and is sung, simply and beautifully, in the hymn, "Jesus Loves Me, This I Know":

The Emperor and the Children

Jesus loves me! This I know,
For the Bible tells me so;
Little ones to Him belong;
They are weak, but He is strong.

Yes, Jesus loves me!
Yes, Jesus loves me!
Yes, Jesus loves me!
The Bible tells me so.

Jesus loves me! This I know,
As He loved so long ago,
Taking children on His knee,
Saying, "Let them come to Me."

Jesus loves me still today,
Walking with me on my way,
Wanting as a friend to give
Light and love to all who live.

Jesus loves me! He who died
Heaven's gate to open wide;
He will wash away my sin,
Let His little child come in.

Jesus loves me! He will stay
Close beside me all the way;
Thou hast bled and died for me,
I will henceforth live for Thee.

Anna B. Warner

Courage through Chronic Disease

Notes

    1. *Return to Tipasa*, 1954, in *The Unquiet Vision: Mirrors of Man in Existentialism*, ed. Nathan A. Scott (New York: World Publishing Company, 1969), 116. Variant translation: "In the depths of winter, I finally learned that within me there lay an invincible summer."

Chapter 7

Grief Revealed

A necessary part of being human is enduring many kinds of grief. They can come at any time and have many causes. As those who have frequently visited the valley of grief can attest, sorrow comes to all. It is often accompanied by severe agony, and feeling better is hard to believe. In time, the agony lessens, but a scar remains. We are changed, but it is possible to be happy again.

Grief is an intrinsic element of a chronic degenerative disease and its subsequent limitations. How this grief is acknowledged and reduced depends on one's personality, coping skills, and use of support systems. Management is distinctive to each person. Dealing with the diagnosis and the decline are also a cause of grief for the person's family and friends.

Death spares no one, sick or healthy, and is the foremost cause of grief. Even when death is expected, it can be upsetting. A major cause of grief is the sudden death of a child.

In his book, *High Wind at Noon* Allan Knight Chalmers tells us about the extraordinary story of Peer Holm. It illustrates the highest response to grief. Peter was a world famous engineer. He built great bridges, railroads, and tunnels in many parts of the world; he gained wealth and fame, but later came to failure, poverty, and sickness. He returned to the little village where he was born and, together with his wife and little girl, eked out a meager living.

> Peer Holm had a neighbor who owned a fierce dog. Peer warned him that the dog was dangerous, but the old man contemptuously replied, "Hold your tongue, you cursed pauper." One day Peer Holm came home to find the dog at the throat of his little girl. He tore the dog away, but the dog's teeth had gone too deeply and the little girl was dead.
>
> The sheriff shot the dog, and the neighbors were bitter against his owner. When sowing time came, they refused to sell him any grain. His fields were plowed but bare. He could neither beg, borrow, nor buy seed. Whenever he walked down the road, the people of the village sneered at him. But not Peer Holm. He could not sleep at night for thinking of his neighbor.
>
> Very early one morning he rose, went to his shed, and got his last half bushel of barley. He climbed the fence and sowed his neighbor's field. The fields themselves told the story. When the seeds came up, it was revealed what Peer had done, because part of his own field remained bare while the field of his neighbor was green.[1]

Peter Holm's response to his daughter's sudden death was extraordinary. He exemplified goodness amid the greatest grief a person can endure.

Grief Revealed

The grief of disease takes place through losses in health, such as incontinence, amputation, lesions, or deformity, and losses in social standing, such as losing a job, being dependent on others for daily needs, decreased financial resources, or elimination of future plans. Specific activities related to grief can be stumbling blocks or stepping stones. Examples of blocks are hyperactivity, excessive sleeping and eating, drinking alcoholic beverages, drug addiction, or anything that prevents the restoration of life energies.

Steps forward include family members and good friends who help meet the challenges of loss, pursuing an educational goal or a new hobby, interest, social activity, or religious practice. The difficulty of moving through grief can be helped by comforts from unexpected sources. A book, poem, song, and supportive people lighten the load and direct our path. As the certainty of loss settles in, we face its reality, grow with its sorrow, and get on with our lives. If we do not face the pain of loss, somewhere it will wait for us. We must go through it to move ahead.

Because disease grief is often overlooked, we may have it and not realize it. Signs could be wanting to be alone, an unkempt appearance, prolonged depression, apathy, or excessive mourning about who we were. At diagnosis, or disease recurrence, grief may not be recognized because of denial, camouflage, or unrealistic expectations about getting better.

When acknowledged, attempts at alleviation may be harmful because the grief is so new. After the initial impact, it is beneficial to wait for a sign that indicates grief is loosening its hold. This occurs when an individual can recognize grief, see beyond it, and believe that the passage of time will soften it. Once identified, a variety of emotions can be triggered by grief. They can be familiar or undefined, range from a single feeling to several at a time, and cause confusion or a sense of the unreal. Emotions are a natural reaction to our disease, its limitations, treatment, or prognosis. In time, strong negative emotions subside or, when normal, alternate with positive ones.

There are healthy and unhealthy expressions of grief. Some healthy manifestations are crying, sadness, feeling forlorn, or knowing something treasured is gone. People sometimes express loss in inappropriate ways such as screaming at loved ones, temper tantrums, or breaking things. However, it is wise to control rash impulses and focus on a song, fragrance, phrase, scene, or familiar comment that reminds us of better times. These reflections are calming and make it easier to smile at the amusing events of today.

Let the Tears Fall

A small loss can cause unexpected grief. Tears can well up and flow for no apparent reason. Shedding tears as a response to test anxiety, diagnosis, treatment, managing a life-long disease, and even anticipated death, is common and often therapeutic. Tears are purifying; after a cry we look up, relieved and attentive. Tears cleanse, and thereby provide clearer vision. The stress of the moment is eased. Tears are helpful; they can dilute negative feelings, release pent-up stress, purge pessimism, remove unidentifiable anxiety, and generally help us feel better. We need not be ashamed of crying, nor be surprised that a smile can break through the tears. We smile as we are revitalized to do our best with the cards we have been dealt. Moreover, with that smile, a new chapter in our book of life can begin.

Other disease grief factors that may need to be addressed are extreme long-term responses to a specific loss, such as the need to use adaptive equipment; unforgiven, unresolved, or harsh feelings; conflicts caused by the disease or aspects of its treatment; or a strong negative reaction when regular care is changed to palliative care. It is not unusual for someone to burst into tears when trying to solve the seemingly endless problems associated with a chronic disease.

At times, grief can evolve into a heart-moving action. Thomas Dorsey was an American musician and composer who lived in Chicago, Illinois. In 1932, his wife Nettie died while giving birth to their son. The baby died the next day. Thomas Dorsey's grief was inconsolable. Yet it inspired him to write what was to become a time-honored classic hymn. The words reflect what people feel when everything seems to be going wrong:

> Precious Lord, take my hand, lead me on, let me stand,
> I am tired, I am weak, I am worn.
> Through the storm, through the night, lead me on to the light.
> Take my hand, precious Lord, lead me home.[2]

Grief as a Channel for Growth

Grief handled well can be a start-up for psychological, social, and spiritual growth. Although our initial response to grief interferes with growth, in time we learn to let go of what grieves us and concentrate on positive things that enhance our sense of value and purpose. When grief agitates us, it can be mitigated by doing soothing tasks that produce a feeling of composure, such as working on a patchwork quilt, making a birdhouse out of wood, or planning a project for a relative.

Grief can offer positive bonding when friends, family, or a support group give encouragement, practical suggestions, comfort, guidance, and prayer. If our grief is excessive, remains the same, or increases, we need to consult a grief counselor, therapist, or member of the clergy who can offer appropriate techniques to keep the grief in check and assist with related issues, such as the inability to make decisions or constant self-defeating thoughts.

An established daily routine helps us stay in the present, reconnect with familiar people, ordinary activities, and current events. Activities such as listening to soothing music, walking the dog, cleaning the kitchen, relaxing with a cup of tea, or doing anything that refreshes and revitalizes gives structure to our days, purpose for our time, and a sense of normalcy.

Henri Nouwen advises:

> You live all these passages in an environment where you are constantly tempted to be destroyed by resentment, by anger, and by a feeling of being put down. The losses remind you constantly that all isn't perfect and it doesn't always happen for you the way you expected; that perhaps you had hoped events would not have been so painful, but they were; or that you expected something from certain relationships that never materialized. You find yourself disillusioned with the irrevocable personal losses: your health, … your job, your hope, your dream. Your whole life is filled with losses, endless losses. And every time there are losses, there are choices to be made. You choose to live your losses as passages

to anger, blame, hatred, depression, and resentment, or you choose to let these losses be passages to something new, something wider, and deeper. The question is not how to avoid loss and make it not happen, but how to choose it as a passage, as an exodus to greater life and freedom.[3]

When we find positive elements in our grief, it leads to a deeper life experience. Feeling sad about what has been lost in the past is replaced by the prospect of finding constructive possibilities in the future. Well channeled, grief is an invitation to love another person, a good cause or a needed service, as well as to develop the powers of the mind, heart, and soul.

Memento Mori: Remember You Must Die

External customs and signs of mourning visualize grief. For those of us who are older, how can we forget the horse-drawn caisson, the muffled drums, and the riderless horse during the funeral of President John F. Kennedy? In the past, these mourning practices were more common than they are today. Black-bordered letters or envelopes, black armbands and ribbons, dark ribbons on a large wreath on the front door, or wearing dark clothes for a period of time were practices that reminded us of the deceased loved one.

Today police wear a small black band on their badges in remembrance of a fallen officer, or members of sport teams wear black arm-bands in memory of a fellow athlete. Roadside memorials are erected at the site where people died in the street. Personal practices include placing a flower by a deceased loved one's picture, lighting a candle to honor a person's memory, or if we are Catholic, a request that a Mass be celebrated on the anniversary of a loved one's death. Expressions of mourning soothe grief. Although it decreases, we rarely get over great losses. They change us. By saying "yes" to grace, and with ongoing determination, these changes can be pleasing to God and help us to cultivate a greater compassion toward the needs of others.

Great grief due to a loved one's death heightens our vulnerability, which needs to be protected. We should avoid making major decisions, such as changing a job, buying a new car or other major purchases, or making a move, until grief has dissipated. Big changes based on impulse or emotion during a grieving period can do more harm than good. Because the loss is so raw, clichés like "be strong," "he is out of his misery," or "he is in a better place," although well intended, usually do not help. When we meet someone who has lost a dear one, it is best to acknowledge his or her loss with simple words. Great grief, like great beauty, may be too deep for words.

> Nothing can make up for the absence of someone whom we love, and it would be wrong to try to find a substitute. That sounds very hard at first, but at the same time, it is a great consolation. For the gap, as long as it remains unfilled, preserves the bond between us. It is nonsense to say that God fills the gap: he doesn't fill it, but on the contrary, he keeps it empty and so helps us to keep alive our former communion with each other, even at the cost of pain. The dearer and richer our memories, the more difficult the separation, but gratitude changes the pangs of memory into a tranquil joy. We must take care not to wallow in our memories, or hand ourselves over to them. Just as we do not gaze all the time at a

valuable present, but only at special times, and apart from these keep it simply as a hidden treasure that is ours for certain.

Dietrich Bonhoeffer [4]

Light at the End of the Tunnel

Light shines on us in many ways. Psalm 34:18 affirms, "The Lord is near to the brokenhearted and saves the crushed in spirit." Mary is a beacon in our sorrow. Many women share in Mary's suffering, but no woman equals her in the depths of her pain. She was young when death snatched her beloved husband from her. She stood by her Son when he was tortured and crucified. It is impossible to imagine her anguish, yet her untold pain never turned to bitterness against those who were responsible for Jesus' death. Her universal motherhood embraces all humanity, from those she knows to far-flung strangers who do not know her Son. As she gently leads us to Jesus, her motherly gaze inscribes on our heart that we are loved by the Lord and will never be abandoned by him.

After someone dear to us dies, it takes a rare kind of courage, and grace, to stop asking, "Why?" At that point, we move past the questions and begin to pick up the pieces. As time passes, the grief of loss can change us into a better Christian. We let go of the hurt and anger that developed from feeling deserted by a loved one, and let his or her memory open our heart to understanding and a hope that is available in no other way. Love never ends and is greater than death. A loved one comes from God, and at death, returns to God, as we will when our time comes.

What can we do to adjust after the one we loved is no longer physically with us? We can set aside a few moments each day to think deeply about the dear one, write a letter or poem to him or her, plant a tree, start a garden, establish a scholarship or memorial fund, or donate books, money, or other life-sustaining items in memory of the loved one. Many fine organizations were founded because of the death of a dear one.

Life's journey unfolds times of grief and joy. Both are necessary to expand the heart, mind, and soul. Joy is an expression of love. It gives our lives special moments of delight, unites people, and brings pleasure to our days. Sorrow can evolve into joy if we allow it. Sorrow breaks our heart, but with grace it mends; it darkens our mind, but dawns with insights that enlighten and inform; it drains energy, but is recharged by new hope. Joy does not disappear when sorrow abounds. It lies unnoticed below the sorrow and emerges when the darkness dissipates. Psalm 30:5 says, "Weeping may tarry for the night, but joy comes with the morning."

How can one grieve if one has not loved? Grief and love are related. Both weave into the tapestry of life. Poor is the person who has not grieved. Those who have been hammered, filed, and tempered in the furnace of grief experience the beauty, joy, and enhancement of life in the garden of love. Happy are those who grieve, for their love has been well spent.

May the Divine Assistance Remain with Us

A reaction to having a chronic disease, or to the death of a loved one, can initiate hostility toward God, or ambivalence and doubts about religion. Sudden sorrow may cause us to lash out at God, but we need not fear his response. He knows our anger even before we do. Conversely, our response

Grief Revealed

to divine love may motivate us to return to the religion of our childhood, or renew our spiritual journey. Renewal can start or restart at any point in life, and reveal talents previously unknown.

Joseph Scriven was poor. He lived in Canada, so he could not visit his mother in Ireland when she became very ill. Instead, he sent her a comforting letter and enclosed a poem he wrote. The simple poem came from his heart. It became a beloved hymn:

> What a friend we have in Jesus, all our sins and griefs to bear.
> What a privilege to carry, everything to God in prayer.
> Oh what peace we often forfeit, oh what needless pain we bear.
> All because we do not carry, everything to God in prayer.[5]

We are encouraged to share our sorrows with Jesus. He is our refuge and our strength. In Matt. 11:28, Jesus said, "Come to me, all you who labor and are heavy laden, and I will give you rest." Moreover, in Matt. 5:4, Jesus said, "Blessed are those who mourn, for they shall be comforted."

The reaction to grief can increase our awareness of God and strengthen faith, as it did with Joseph Scriven. We discover strength in forgiveness, hope in failure, and security in faith. Jesus said, "Let not your hearts be troubled neither let them be afraid. Peace I leave with you, my peace I give to you; not as the world gives do I give to you" (John 14:27).

Integrating loss is a slow and difficult process. We rely on God in ways we can never imagine. The assurance that God is in control sustains us with grace that enables us to live with paradox, conflict, and unanswered questions. We look deeper into what we believe and find treasures beyond this valley of tears. Faith is a gift that must be received, opened, and lived each day. Whether our faith seems weak or strong, we stick with it and tend to our daily spiritual practices.

As we accept our disease and mortality, life becomes enriched and profound. Trust in God helps us beyond description. It is only in God and through God that we can fully experience ourselves as authentic human beings. 2 Corinthians 1:3–4 tells us: "Blessed be the God and Father of our Lord Jesus Christ, the Father of mercies and God of all comfort, who comforts us in all our affliction, so that we may be able to comfort those who are in any affliction, with the comfort with which we ourselves are comforted by God."

> Be still, sad heart and cease repining;
> Behind the clouds is the sun still shining;
> Thy fate is the common fate of all,
> Into each life some rain must fall.
> Henry Wadsworth Longfellow[6]

Notes

1. Charles Allen, *God's Psychiatry* (Ada, MI: Fleming H. Revell Company 1953), 146–147.

2. For full lyrics: https://aaregistry.org/poem/take-my-hand-precious-lord-by-thomas-a-dorsey/.

3. https://henrinouwen.org/meditations/passages-to-new-life/.

4. Holy card created by the Discalced Carmelite nuns, Monastery of St. Joseph, Port Tobacco, MD. https://www.carmelofporttobacco.com Quote: https://legacy.npr.org/programs/death/readings/spiritual

Grief Revealed

/bonh.html#:~:text=Nothing%20can%20make%20up%20for, preserves%20the%20bonds%20between%20us.

5. For full lyrics: https://www.hymnal.net/en/hymn/h/789.

6. Henry Wadsworth Longfellow, "The Rainy Day." For complete poem: see Bartleby.com, 780. The Rainy Day, from English Poetry III: From Tennyson to Whitman, *The Harvard Classics*. 1909–14, https://www.bartleby.com/42/780.html.

Chapter 8

Adjustments on the Road

One of the most difficult aspects of living with a chronic disease is adapting everyday life to one's new limitations. We see examples in many who have been diagnosed with polio. Polio, also known as poliomyelitis or infantile paralysis, is an infectious viral disease that inflames the brain and spinal cord and, when severe, can lead to muscle wasting and loss of voluntary movement. During the late 1940s, polio outbreaks in the United States increased in frequency and size, disabling an average of more than 35,000 people each year.[1] 1952 was the worst polio year on record with more than 57,000 cases nationwide.[2] It was one of the most feared diseases of the twentieth century. It came without warning to people of any age and required long quarantines. The consequences of the disease left people using wheelchairs, crutches, leg braces, breathing devices, and the most remembered: the iron lung.

Post-polio syndrome affects between twenty-five and forty out of every one hundred polio survivors. It starts about fifteen to forty years after the initial infection.[3] Common symptoms are a gradual weakness and decrease in size of muscles that were previously affected by polio, muscle and joint pain, and mental and physical fatigue. Its symptoms can make it difficult for a person to function independently. Don contracted this disease. His wife, Pauline, reflects:

> I met my husband when I was twenty years old. We had an old-fashioned courtship and were married in 1970. Don was an exceptional person and I have many fond memories of our forty-four years together. My life has been greatly blessed by a wonderful husband and three lively children.
>
> When Don was eighteen months old, he contracted polio. His mother saw his right arm shrivel up so fast it gave her the fright of her life. Don had limitations from his polio for the rest his life. However, they did not stop him. The very first credit goes to his mother regarding his attitude toward it. She didn't baby him and expected him to do things any of her other kids did. Too many mothers baby their kids when they have a problem.
>
> Don had a positive outlook that lasted throughout his life. When he was in high school, he wanted to join the track team and some other sports team but in the late fifties and early sixties they didn't have the Americans with Disabilities Act as they do now, so both team coaches said they were afraid that he would get hurt. So he became the manager of both teams instead. He loved being manager and was proud of earning the school letters.
>
> Like other married couples, we had our arguments, but Don never lost his temper with me. He was a kind but firm disciplinarian with our kids. They admired and respected their dad. When there were some small problems concerning the limitations caused by the polio, we would figure out how to go around or work with them.

Adjustments on the Road

For example, when our oldest child was a baby, Don could not pin her diaper (this was before Pampers). So we found a pair of rubber pants that used a diaper liner which worked out fine. This seems like a small problem but it illustrates the many times we found other ways to go around some difficulty. Don worked as a dispatcher and assistant manager for a truck company and was active in several organizations. In his last years he needed more help. After he passed away, I talked with several people and realized what a blessing it was that he did not resent the help he received from others when he needed it. It made helping him very easy. He did not give up, which I saw others do.

As the years pass, I realize more and more what a special person Don was.[4]

Don was resilient and lived his life with a beautiful, positive orientation. He did not think about the things polio prevented him from doing, but concentrated on what he could do and did them well.

Winding Roads and Wind Storms

The road of life is full of countless curves and detours that can lead to unknown or unwelcome destinations. Sometimes they come slowly, sometimes in rapid succession. Traveling around unexpected bends or on rough roads is a never-ending and intimidating part of life. Big or small, changes are inevitable. Each adjustment is different, unique to the situation and the person dealing with it. Sometimes it seems like we are in a strange land. We lose our naiveté. We may have thought we would never get this particular disease. However, we got it and it can bring innumerable adjustments.

Courage through Chronic Disease

During diagnostic testing or in early disease stages we may feel like trees in a windstorm. We may be trees with shallow roots or with deep roots. Oak trees are beautiful and seem strong and hardy. However, because of their shallow root system they can fall by strong winds. Pine trees are as beautiful as oak trees. Their roots are deep and they remain standing in a storm. In the same way, shallowly rooted people are easily toppled by the strong winds of a disease. They fall over and remain in their heap of misery because they depend on circumstances to make them happy. Deeply rooted people know happiness comes from within. They are at risk, but their roots keep them anchored when storm winds blow. Roots matter. If they are deep in the truths and laws of God, they sustain character, and initiate graces that make ongoing adjustments to a degenerative disease constructive and easier to bear. When strong winds from a serious disease come, the individual remains steadfast in hope and faith, and takes bad weather in stride. Disease is not a punishment from God for bad behavior, the devil's curse, or something a person deserves for whatever reason. If new health concerns are put into perspective, they become another part of an individual and life moves on. Upheavals from chronic diseases pass. Indeed, roots deepen when fierce winds blow.

Suffering cannot be avoided; therefore, it is best to keep it as positive as we can. Teresa of Calcutta reminds us that suffering will never be absent from our lives. We should not be afraid of it, because it is a great means of love if we make use of it by offering it for peace in the world. She goes on to say that suffering of itself is useless, but suffering shared with the passion of Christ is a great gift and a sign of love. During her life, Teresa of Calcutta saw profound human suffering and lived in deep faith. She knew that faith means the courage to live with uncertainty. It does not mean having the answers, but rather the courage to ask the questions and not let go of God, since he will not let go of us. She realized that God creates divine justice, and all of us, who act in accord with his word, can create human justice. This is God's will for us. He sees the potential for goodness and holiness in each of us, and as reflections of his goodness, we care for others.

A serious chronic disease can change us for better or for worse. We are responsible for responding appropriately to change. Faith will not allow us to lazily resign ourselves to a chronic condition, ignore it, or deny it. To believe every life is unique and irreplaceable is a sign that we are striving toward well-being. Having a chronic disease does not mean well being is not accessible to us, because it is an integrated concept referring to all areas of human development for which we strive in spite of our physical, mental, or spiritual flaws. A disease can plague our bodies and influence our minds but it cannot touch our souls unless we allow it.

The Importance of Anger Adjustment

Angry feelings can range from irritability to outrage, and are triggered by a number of things: confusion, frustration, hurt, fear, alarm, or a dreaded diagnosis. After diagnosis, almost anything can initiate it: too many sticks for a blood draw, a long hold on the phone when scheduling a test, a very short visit with a health care professional after an extensive wait.

Feeling anger is not the major concern. What we do with it defines us. Appropriate anger does not hurt others, and is expressed in clear and assertive but non-confrontational ways, such as describing the anger problem, rather than blaming, criticizing, or attacking others. Inappropriate anger harms others and us. Ignoring, suppressing, or venting anger in destructive ways is detrimental. Buried anger can fester in the heart for years and manifest as resentment, vengeance, tension, or sarcastic humor. It is dangerous to let anger accumulate because it can explode in the face of unsuspecting dear ones.

There are appropriate ways to defuse anger. It may be impossible to control the situation that caused anger, but we can control how we react to it. Pinpoint the source of the anger, and focus on resolving that issue rather than on the anger surrounding it. Anger can be used to mask feelings of insecurity, resentment, hurt, shame, or fear. If anger expresses these feelings, it can erode growth in genuine faith and trust. Holding on to inappropriate anger from the past, even though what caused the anger may be forgotten, is a heavy weight. We need to release it to be at peace with the past and live in the reality of today. Because anger can fuel negative responses, it needs to be recognized. At the first sign of losing our temper, we can slowly count to ten or twenty before we say anything, take deep breaths, exercise, jog, or stretch areas of muscle tension. We can also take a few minutes to collect our thoughts before speaking. We might even try to find humor in the situation.

An old story may help to rethink our anger issues. On a foggy morning, a farmer gathered his produce and put it in his boat to take it to the market. As he was going upstream, another boat was coming downstream and was directly in the farmer's path. As the boats came closer, the farmer tried to veer away as he shouted, "Get out of the way or else we will collide." His voice grew stronger as his anger increased. When the boats collided, the furious farmer turned to yell at the other boatman. His anger evaporated when he saw that the boat was empty. The boat had just come loose from its mooring. The farmer calmed down and gently pushed the boat away. From that point on, whenever he felt his anger rise at a person, the farmer treated the person like an empty boat.

On the positive side, anger occurs when people care. They express anger when they stand up for what they believe or value. Jesus gives an example of righteous anger in John 2:13–16: "The Passover of the Jews was at hand, and Jesus went up to Jerusalem. In the temple he found those who were selling oxen and sheep and pigeons, and the money-changers at their business. And making a whip of cords, he drove them all, with the sheep and oxen, out of the temple; and he poured out the coins of the money-changers and overturned their tables. And he told those who sold the pigeons, 'Take these things away; you shall not make my Father's house a house of trade.'" Jesus was angry about what was going on in his Father's house, and for a good reason: to restore the temple as a house of God.

When we get angry with a person, or with certain people, we need to step back and reflect. We probably do not know the whole story about what they are going through, what they are thinking, or why they act the way they do. Sometimes we just have to let things go. And for our own sanity, we should never let the sun go down on our anger.

Accept Finite Disappointment, but Do Not Lose Infinite Hope

Living with a serious chronic disease will include innumerable disappointments. We get a negative report from our doctor. We need more treatment. An anticipated visit from a friend does not happen or happens when we are bone tired. Life has many disappointments, and they increase with a chronic disease.

Jesus did not say we would not have hard times. He said he would be with us. When he is present, disappointments are easier as we roll with the punches. Prayer and hope sustain us. Hope is not a naive optimism, but a disposition that accepts challenges and suffering as a part of life. Hope puts all in the hands of God, and helps us to be resilient. Disappointments should never be a mind set or anticipated at every turn. To not fuss over disappointing trifles makes it easier to withstand hard blows. If we lightly accept disappointments as they happen, and balance them by naming joyful events we treasure, it mitigates the disappointments.

For a while, being upset about a disappointment is common, but keeping an indefinite hold on it is depleting. A great gift is to garner an increased capacity to face unpleasantness and disappointments without being unduly upset or morose. With the passing of time, we learn to react calmly to little disappointments. Big disappointments cause inner hurt and confusion; however, they too shall pass. Whatever caused the disappointment may not have been beneficial for us in the long run. We may not have known certain harmful incidences, or have an accurate back story, about the situation that caused the disappointment. Perhaps it protected us from an unknown danger. Let-downs can be like days that begin with a fierce storm and end with a calm evening sky.

A brilliant and financially successful businessman became the father of a developmentally disabled daughter. He wondered why this happened to him. Later he discovered that if he had not had that child he would have pursued a shallow life, lost to the goods and gods of worldly success. She taught him to love.

Change as an Instructor

We tend to our health needs, but they are not our primary identity, nor do we use them to take advantage of others. Once we have done what is necessary, and take reasonable preventive measures, we have done our part. Being preoccupied about our disease, being defined by it, or incessantly talking about it, is self-defeating. We try to avoid unnecessary health care worries, unsolicited advice, or flim-flam treatments. They confuse the mind, and may cause us to withdraw from others. Instead we do our utmost to have confidence in God.

Enduring a chronic condition should increase our reverence for the sacredness of life. It refines the importance of being polite, keeping our word, and living in peace with that which we cannot change. The ability to say, "I was wrong" (and, when we are right, not saying, "I told you so"). "I am sorry," "Forgive me," "Please" and "Thank you" shows courtesy to, and respect for, those with whom we speak. Remaining tranquil in the midst of chaos and disagreeing without being disagreeable can be like an oasis of peace for those with whom we live and others. Living with a long-term physical condition sheds light on things we previously took for granted. We are more conscious of the fragility of life, kind acts from others, laughter of children, fragile beauty of the elderly, birdsong, butterflies, and spiritual practices.

Jesus is our refuge when we are caught in a sea of negativity. He helps us look at, and move toward, the shore of life. If we are psychologically or emotionally numb, we give ourselves a good shake and wake up to the liveliness of the day. When we think we are at the end of our rope, we find consolation in simple prayers such as the beautiful: "Jesus I trust in you."

The Wonder of Journaling

Many famous people, from all walks of life, kept journals or diaries. Among them were Benjamin Franklin, Thomas Edison, Winston Churchill, Mark Twain, Christopher Columbus, and Lewis and Clark. In the area of spirituality, personal reflections have become spiritual classics: Teresa of Avila wrote her *Life*, Therese of Lisieux penned *The Story of a Soul*, Faustina of Poland, her *Diary*, and Augustine of Hippo documented his life in the *Confessions*.

However, most journals remain private and are written by ordinary people. Journaling is good therapy in many ways. In an environment filled with external stimuli, it keeps us connected with ourselves. By recording difficulties with our disease, we can reread them after some time and find new insights. Writing can be a rest, or a release from issues that concern us about not being physically normal. As our words unfold, they can shine new light on perplexing situations.

Journaling can be used as a sounding board, a way to reduce mind overload, a means for self-knowledge, or an exercise in creativity. Our words can be sad, sublime, jocular, mysterious, fun, or formal. Contents of a journal offer interior stabilization amid external adjustments due to our disease progression. Recording thoughts, ideas, feelings, opinions, or insights reveals more about who we are than watching TV, surfing the Internet, talking on the phone, or using social media. Regular journaling is a time- honored source for self-discovery.

When Paul was sixteen his uncle died. Paul's predominate memory was his uncle sitting in a wheelchair; he did not remember much else. However, the uncle's journal revealed that he was a man of many parts and well-honed talents. Hearing journal entries expands our perception and appreciation of another person. Journaling can serve as a means for guidance, goals, self-exploration, personal struggles, frustrations, and achievements. Most importantly it can be a spiritual diary. Paul had no idea his uncle's favorite prayer was the Memorare.[5]

A pen and sturdy three-ring binder with removable pages, and tabs that identify reflection topics can serve us well. Titles identify any area that is significant to us and might include: rites of passage, fond memories, literary selections, or limericks. Negatives, like stresses, problems, or challenges, are balanced by positives, such as solutions, joys, or resolutions. A most important tab is spirituality. It connects us with eternal life, and may contain favorite verses from holy books, cherished prayers, and reflections. Everyone has words of wisdom, but we may assume that we cannot write. However, how do we really know unless we give it a try?

Entries can range from deep thoughts to silly ruminations, it doesn't matter what we write. Unless we desire it, there will be no one to edit, censor, or correct our efforts.

Our writing style is distinctly our own. We do not have to be profound or meaningful. A journal is only for us to see, or, if we desire, to share with someone.

How much journaling should be dedicated to our disease experience? Short or long, the choice is ours. We could write about our disease concerns, uncertainties about the future, woes, or rages. If we write thoughts or feelings that are deeply troubling, we need help and tell them to a trusted and wise person. We could draw something that represents our disease, or write down words of a theme song for our journey. The entertainer Jerry Lewis used to close his muscular dystrophy telethons with the song, "When you walk through a storm, hold your head up high, and don't be afraid of the dark. . . ."

It is best to write in a quiet environment where there are no interruptions. We try to relax and be calm as we focus on a particular theme. Dates and times for entries depend on us. The constant is that we date each entry and remain faithful to this practice, be it weekly or monthly. Since each person perceives an event differently, we write about our perception of an event rather than the event itself. Sorted out and expressed on paper, writing can be a cathartic release for a jumble of negative thoughts. Use of metaphors, or pen names instead of names of people who irritate us are helpful. Writing can soften and clear our inner landscape, removing negative thoughts that clutter the mind or drain energy. Over time, we may notice changes in our patterns of thinking and behavior, as we learn what is below the surface of our routine reactions.

A journal is very personal and needs to be kept in a safe place away from prying eyes. If we write hurtful letters to those who have caused us anger, grief, or resentment, after a few days we remove and destroy them. We could use a word processor for journaling, but that is more public, as is writing on a web site. The internet is considered public so anything written on it can resemble a personal editorial and should be composed with that in mind. The process of writing with a pen rather than a keyboard is considered a more satisfying therapeutic practice for journaling.

Where would we be without the written word? If we fear taking pen in hand, we only need to look at the Bible. The Bible reveals God's presence and activities in the lives of people. The epistles are ten percent of Bible contents. These letters are presented in a concise and organized format. The rest is eclectic in its writing styles and contains a wide range of topics such as incredible stories, high drama, epic history, meditative poetry, and homespun parables. Events in the Gospels are written in different ways. Continuums of faith, doubt, good and evil, flow through its pages. Yet, has any other book changed so many lives and lifestyles?

Different Ways of Winning

Before our chronic disease, we may have thought that winning meant receiving a first place trophy. The tough days of our disease teach us that winning means running the course through a variety of ways, such as completing a difficult diagnostic test, undergoing that needed surgery, finishing a phase of treatment, doing something we were afraid of doing, or learning something new. Winning can be smiling when people say they are proud of us, accomplishing a goal we set for ourselves, overcoming a problem, or being happy for someone else who has won. On the home front, needed things that have been procrastinated because they cause anxiety or fear, such as making a doctor's appointment or having a diagnostic test are completed. After we do it, we feel relief and renewed courage, a win score for the day. We overcame a fear and we can do it again. Experience tells us that imagined fears are usually greater than the real fear. Fear is like being in a dense, damp fog. However, soon the sun burns away that fog and all is bright again. Life's journey is made up of small steps of courage. Within a chronic affliction, those small steps broaden our perspective of winning.

Changes from a chronic disease close some doors and open others. Openings are new beginnings, or creative opportunities, that keep us moving forward. We work with what we have, respect our limits, and discover innovative courses of action. Something once learned can be learned again at a new and deeper level. Itzhak Perlman, the legendary violinist, uses crutches due to polio. In autumn of 1995, when he was performing onstage at the Lincoln Center a string popped. Perlman recomposed the piece in his head and new beautiful sounds never heard before came from the remaining three strings of his violin. He knew that it is the task of musicians to find out how much music they can still make with what they have left. Chronic disease can break our strings, but what treasures are released through these breaks?

Broken strings on the physical level may mean stronger strings on the spiritual level. A sound spiritual orientation and prayerful practices are unequalled helps in adjusting to the curves and detours of life. The graces of loving and learning about God can be very simple. When we want to learn more about God, what comes to mind?

Adjustments on the Road

What hast thou learnt today?
Hast thou sounded awful mysteries,
Hast pierced the veiled skies,
Climbed to the feet of God,
Trodden where saints have trod,
Fathomed the heights above?
Nay,
This only have I learnt, that God is love.

What hast thou heard today?
Hast heard the angel trumpets cry,
And rippling harps reply;

Heard from the throne of flame
Whence God incarnate came
Some thunderous message roll?
Nay,
This have I heard, His voice within my soul.

What hast thou felt today?
The pinions of the angel guide
That standeth at thy side
In rapturous ardours beat,
Glowing, from head to feet,
In ecstasy divine?
Nay,
This only have I felt, Christ's hand in mine.

Robert Hugh Benson[6]

Notes

1. National Center for Immunization and Respiratoory Diseases, (NCIRD) Division of Viral Dieases, "Polio in the United States," https://www.cdc.gov/polio/what-is-polio/polio-us.html.

2. David M. Oshinsky, *Polio: An American Story* (New York, NY: Oxford University Press, 2005), 160.

3. National Center for Immunization and Respiratoory Diseases, (NCIRD) Division of Viral Dieases, "Post-Polio Syndrome," https://www.cdc.gov/polio/what-is-polio/pps.html.

4. Author's conversation with Pauline Chapnan, December 15, 2022.

5. Remember, O most gracious Virgin Mary, that never was it known that anyone who fled to thy protection, implored thy help, or sought thy intercession, was left unaided. Inspired by this confidence I fly unto thee, O Virgin of virgins, my mother. To thee do I come, before thee I stand, sinful and sorrowful. O Mother of the Word Incarnate, despise not my petitions, but in thy mercy hear and answer me. Amen. Biblioteca Apostiolica Vaticana, "The Memorare," https://www.vaticannews.va/en/prayers/the-memorare.html.

6. Kenneth Christopher, ed., *A Sampler of Devotional Poems* (Mahwah, NJ: Paulist Press, 1997), 56–57.

Chapter 9

Perseverance as the Motivator

When Thomas Carlyle had finished the first volume of his book *The French Revolution*, he gave the finished manuscript to his friend John Stuart Mill and asked him to read it. It took Mr. Mill several days to read it and as he read, he realized that it was truly a great literary achievement. Late one night as he finished the last page, he laid the manuscript aside by his chair in the den of his home. The next morning the maid came. Seeing those papers on the floor, she thought they were simply discarded; she threw them into the fire, and they were burned.

On March 6, 1835—he never forgot the date—Mill called on Carlyle in deep agony and told him that his work had been destroyed. Carlyle replied, "It's all right. I'm sure I can start over in the morning and do it again."

Finally, after great apologies, John Mill left and started back home. Carlyle watched his friend walking away and said to his wife, "Poor Mill, I feel so sorry for him. I did not want him to see how crushed I really am." Then heaving a sigh, he said, "Well, the manuscript is gone, so I had better start writing again."

> It was a long, hard process especially because the inspiration was gone. It is always hard to recapture the verve and the vigor if a man has to do a thing like that twice. But he set out to do it again and finally completed the work.
>
> Thomas Carlyle walked away from disappointment. He could do nothing about a manuscript that was burned up. So it is with us: There are times to get up and get going and let what hapened happen.[1]

For a long-term project like writing a book, a vision is needed before one begins. Thomas Carlyle had that vision. A person who is serious about wholistic well-being should have a vision that would make this world a better place. Long-term health conditions have taught us that difficult times can open us to a deeper awareness of what is going on around us. Our chronic disease struggles help us to understand the struggles of others.

Everyone needs a vision, a sound, believable dream. Motivation, partnered by perseverance, creates the incentive to do things to realize that vision. We ask, what do I want to create, build, shape, or share? We may notice a need because of our physical limitations. After we define it, we act according to our beliefs, talents, and wisdom. Perseverance moves us forward with direction and purpose.

Minor visions are just as important as major ones. Chronic health issues lead to several minor visions: positive thinking when facing weary and discouraging circumstances, making it through the day, or treatment, and most importantly getting up after being knocked down by an exacerbation, complication, or setback. Managing a chronic disease

Preserverance as the Motivator

proves that anything worthwhile requires hard work and determination.

Positive motivation is the fuel that keeps us moving, as it stimulates creating and doing. Motivation continues when we maintain a measured pace, thus avoiding burnout or rust-out. How free time is spent reveals an individual's motivational level. To desire a better tomorrow is praiseworthy, and should be the motivator to do good today. Proper motivation keeps impetuousness in check, and challenges us to live with problems until they are solved or removed. Perseverance keeps expectations reasonable and offers an alert, forward-thinking orientation until a goal is achieved, changed, or abandoned. There may be changes in our vision if a goal takes on new dimensions or has deepened in meaning with the passing of time.

Delay does not mean something will not happen. Perhaps the time is just not right. We find new information and integrate new life experiences. An unexpected hospitalization, for example, can teach us many things. We are stretched and reshaped into greater maturity and better ability to meet challenges. Learning a skill, mastering a craft, or creating a work of art takes us from being a passive patient to an active creator. At the end, it is more about who we have become while realizing our vision than what we have achieved by the reality of that vision.

Achieving the Objective

A vision without a plan is only wishful thinking, a fanciful inclination, or a passing wonder. We cannot get where we want to go without a specific road map. Perseverance dissolves if we wander around in circles, or have endless excuses about not being able to bring a vision into reality. Calling ourselves demeaning terms causes mental deflation that halts or delays starting work on our vision. Perseverance plows through hesitancies and excuses. If we are serious about our vision, we will develop the talents it takes and find the time it requires. Writing down a realistic vision and goal, within a time frame, clarifies it. Then we record ways to obtain it. We desire to increase our stamina within three months by appropriate exercises for twenty minutes, twice a day. We want to lose one pound every two weeks for five months; no sweets until this happens. If we want to stop excessive talking about our ailments, we read books about conversation skills and watch TV programs and DVDs on the art of dialogue. Then we live what we learned. The path from self-centered conversation may be slow, but people will notice. As we see progress, gratitude for little things along the way brings the vision closer to reality.

To build a better world can be done in simple ways that uplift, educate, and inspire. A few encouraging words can lighten hard work. Cleaning a stuffed closet reveals unneeded items to give away. Teaching in a religious education program builds a spiritual foundation for the students. Looking at pictures painted by foot and mouth artists uplifts and inspires. A positive vision helps us look forward to an activity or creating something better than what is at present. It is also a source to which we return for refreshment and rejuvenation.

A difficult part of dealing with permanent disease is to sustain the perseverance needed to continue with treatment. After a long round of different medications, several surgeries, therapy day after day, or one kind of treatment following another, we may feel so worn out we lose the desire to continue treatment. We may feel disillusioned, depressed, wiped out, or just want to give up or die. At this point, we need to talk with someone who has been there, or a specialized health care professional. Even though we feel abandoned or isolated in our suffering, we are not alone. Sharing our feelings with trusted others can divide our sorrow. There are many low points during treatment and several types of help available. We just have to find the right one. A few words of support from someone who really listens may be just what we need. A smile or friendly greeting from a health care person, or even a stranger, can brighten our day. A positive turning point may come if we experience a burning irritation toward our disease. It can be the energy that starts us up again and keeps us going. We stand firm against what is trying to take us down. In the depths of desperation, we can believe that, at the end of the road, all will be well.

Perseverance is the enthusiasm behind cultivating the soil once a seed has been planted so the seed can grow, or chipping away at a block of stone so that a statue emerges, or painting on a blank canvas to create a beautiful scene. Just as the little acorn grows into a great oak tree, so can a vision become a reality.

An Exemplary Life

Individuals with a chronic disease need to surround themselves with a few people who are a positive and inspirational influence. They give us the push we need to take the next step, and do what we never thought possible.

Courage through Chronic Disease

For countless numbers of people, Helen Keller was an influential, highly motivated person. She was born on June 27, 1880, in Tuscumbia, Alabama. She was physically healthy until the age of nineteen months, when she contracted what seemed to be scarlet fever and lost her hearing and sight. As she grew into childhood, she developed an unruly temper and became unmanageable. In 1887, her parents, Arthur and Kate Keller, contacted the Perkins Institute for the Blind in Boston for a teacher. They hired Anne Sullivan, herself visually impaired, who came to their home.

Anne taught Helen how to read and write in Braille and how to use hand signals to understand and communicate with others. This was illustrated in the Pulitzer Prize winning play, and subsequent movie, The Miracle Worker. With Anne transferring the lectures into Helen's hand, Helen graduated with a Bachelor of Arts degree, *cum laude*, from Radcliffe College in 1904. During her junior year at Radcliffe, she wrote her first book, *The Story of My Life*, which is still in print and translated into over fifty languages. Helen wrote other books about her personal experiences, religion, contemporary social problems, her travels, and a biography of Anne Sullivan. She wrote many articles for national magazines and newspapers about concerns of the blind, the underprivileged, worker's rights, women's suffrage, and other causes.

In 1924 she joined the staff of the newly formed American Foundation for the Blind and served as an adviser, fundraiser, and in other capacities for over forty years. Helen had a warm personality and was well traveled. She was outspoken about her convictions, all of which contributed to her international popularity. Her impact as an educator, advocate, organizer, lecturer, political activist, writer, and fundraiser was enormous. She was responsible for many advances in public services to the deaf and blind and other causes. Helen was widely honored throughout the world, received honorary doctoral degrees, and had invitations to the White House by every president from Grover Cleveland to Lyndon Johnson. Her courage, intelligence, and dedication made her a symbol of faith and strength through adversity.

She sustained a stroke in 1960 and lived quietly at her home until her death on June 1, 1968. At her memorial service, Senator Lister Hill of Alabama said, "She will live on, one of the few, the immortal names not born to die. Her spirit will endure as long as man can read and stories can be told of the woman who showed the world there are no boundaries to courage and faith."[2]

On the Home Front

A sound family has a good spiritual foundation that guides familial interactions. A family member with a chronic disease affects family interactions from positive to negative. That member's reaction to her pain may be misdirected as a verbal blast at another member. This is the pain talking, not the person, and can happen with frustration, depression, or other secondary disease conditions. Patience helps take the blast in stride, forgives easily, and hopes good will develops from the troublesome situation. Perseverance helps bypass the feelings at the moment and concentrates on the commitment to family life.

Everyone has flaws. We may have a relative who is a chronic complainer. Whenever we meet there is always an argument. It is a fight, with the same words and accusations. This scene must change. We choose silence instead of repeated negative responses. We look at our relative and do not repeat anything that was said before. We pause in silence, put ourselves in the other person's shoes, and imagine what he or she may be thinking. Then we say something consoling. For instance, "Even though we don't agree, I love you." This allows us to step away from the bickering and listen to the other person. Arguments fuel flames rather than settle issues. If we are so intent about proving our point, we do not hear the other person. Love can overcome heated arguments, painful encounters, and other inflammatory issues common in family interactions.

When we persevere, we stay on track and keep on moving. It is best to proceed with a sustained, even enthusiasm like rowers in a boat. We continue rowing through calm or troubled water, gently, at times merrily, but mostly consistently. We row our boat because we know where we want to go. We don't try to row other people's boats or let them row ours. In the current of life each of us is responsible for guiding his or her own boat.

Even if we come from an environment that hurts us or weighs us down, we can rise above it and build the fruitful future of our vision. When he was a teen, Robert developed a heart condition. His parents told him he would never amount to anything. Instead of believing them, he proved them wrong. He earned a PhD and became a respected professor. When she was five years old, Julia contracted juvenile insulin dependent diabetes. She managed it well and had compassion for poor children. She went to college, became a social worker, and they were her specialty. Because Michael remembered the crime-infested neighborhood of his youth, and used a wheelchair because of it, he became a probation officer. These goals could not be attained without self-discipline in keeping medical appointments, taking medications, diet, exercise, hygiene, and related areas. Discipline is the bedrock of living with a chronic disease.

Conscience as a Moral Guide

A necessary component for a good conscience is discipline. Discipline makes use of time more efficiently by setting appropriate priorities based on what we can accomplish. It strengthens us to do things we don't want to do. If we did not have the discipline to deal with the rigors of treatment, we would probably no longer be here. Self-mastery strengthens good habits, promotes a healthy respect for others, and sustains a higher standard of living. We examine ourselves, strive to bring out the best in others, and acknowledge and work with our problems. A clear head and calm manner are byproducts of self-mastery. What we do is completed in a deliberate, conscientious, consistent style. When we complete tasks one at a time, it allows us to enjoy the process in doing the task and minimizes the feeling of being swamped or overwhelmed.

On our journey with a chronic condition, there will be many times when we have to make decisions with no easy answers. Our conscience is the major force in choosing what is good or bad for us. An informed conscience gives us the impetus to make the right decisions, even when they are frightening beyond words. Conscience is our moral guide. It is the sense of right and wrong that influences our thoughts, words, and conduct. A well-informed conscience distinguishes what is good and right from that which will harm us. It plays a major role in forming our vision, establishing our goals, and persevering through the complicated and confusing aspects of the health care industry. We obtain information about aspects in the health care system as needed, pray about it, processes it through our intellect, and then, through our will, we decide on a course of action.

An enlightened conscience develops good habits by choices made: holding our tongue here, helping another person there, caring for new symptoms when they appear. The more often we make these choices, the more readily they become our second nature. If we make a decision to read a chapter of the Bible each day, it can become as natural as eating breakfast in the morning. To stick with good health habits has bodily benefits. To maintain spiritual practices is exercise for the soul.

Trust in Divine Guidance

We must trust God to help us deal with our fears and doubts. Even though we lack motivation to make follow-up visits with medical professionals, or undergo specific treatments, we do it anyway because it is the right thing to do. Because we are committed to ongoing medical responsibilities, we do not rely on our feelings to motivate us. If we did, we would easily make excuses and stay home. At times, we may not feel like going, or have the heart for such a visit, but we go anyway. From time to time, we experience a sense of satisfaction, but we do not depend on that to motivate us. The most important aspect is that we are steadfast in our visits, and therefore true to our commitment to do what is right.

Preserverance as the Motivator

We must keep asking God for perseverance. Jesus helps us in this quest by keeping us attentive to what is truly important. Perseverance promotes humility that fosters knowledge and appreciates the goodness and providence of God. The shifting sands of desires concerning the self are slowly replaced by the rock-solid wisdom of Jesus' desires for humanity. The ideals of Christianity can be similar to a river that flows away from the consumerist-driven rapids of the present to the hopeful, placid streams of the unity and peace of God. If we want to aim high, the divine and human personification of love, and our best guide for envisioning goals, is Jesus. For people, especially Christians, Jesus' words, "I am the way, and the truth and the life" (John 14:6), capture a deep need: the answer to where our human life is leading. Jesus teaches us the way to live the virtue of love and do good on earth that leads to eternal life in heaven.

We adhere to divine guidance by living Jesus' words to be on the lookout for false prophets. They wear sheep's clothing but underneath they are wolves on the prowl. They are alive today in the form of brilliant people who are ruthless, cult leaders, highly charismatic people, deceiving wellness promoters, and charlatans who promote complimentary or alternative therapies, or instant cures. The Sermon on the Mount includes the golden rule: Treat others the way you would have them treat you. The Sermon on the Mount needs to be inscribed in our hearts because it is so beneficial to humanity. Tolerance, respect, and reverence help contribute to the goodness in humanity. If we strive to look beyond the contempt we feel for certain people, we may see into their hearts. If we pray for our irritators, we will be surprised at who is changed.

Courage through Chronic Disease

It is fortunate that we do not know what lies ahead on our road of life. If we knew how long it would take to fulfill a vision, we might stop trying. The same may be true for disease-related trials and suffering that come along. On the road of frail health we may be emotionally drained, hear dire statistics, feel vulnerable, or get tired. Nevertheless, with God's help and perseverance, we can make it through. Beneath all those afflictions, we hear a chorus singing, "We Shall Overcome." And we do. And we will do it again. There were times when we did not hear the message, but they were still singing, and they will continue to sing when the future looks bleak.

> I've dreamed many dreams that never came true,
> I've seen them vanish at dawn;
> But I've realized enough of my dreams, thank God,
> To make me want to dream on.
>
> I've prayed many prayers when no answer came,
> I've waited patient and long;
> But answers have come to enough of my prayers
> To make me keep praying on.
>
> I've trusted many a friend who failed
> And left me to weep alone;
> But I've found enough of my friends true blue
> To make me keep trusting on.
>
> I've sown many seeds that fell by the way
> For the birds to feed upon;
> But I've held enough golden sheaves in my hand,
> To make me keep sowing on.
>
> I've drained the cup of disappointment and pain,

Preserverance as the Motivator

I've gone many days without song,
But I've sipped enough nectar from the rose of life
To make me want to live on.³

Ron DeMarco

Notes

1. Adapted from William Barclay, *The King and the Kingdom* (Edinburgh: The Saint Andrew Press, 1969), 161.

2. Eulogy delivered by Senator Lister Hill at the Memorial Service for Miss Helen Keller, Washington Cathedral, Washington, D.C., June 5, 1968: https://www.afb.org/HelenKellerArchive?a=d&d=A-HK01-01-B003-F09-028&e=-------en-20--1--txt--------3-7-6-5-3------------French%2C+R.+S.--0-1≥

3. Shivpreet Singh, "I've Dreamed Many Dreams - Ron Demarco," October 7, 2021, https://www.shivpreetsingh.com/2021/10/ive-dreamed-many-dreams-ron-demarco.html.

Chapter 10

The Essential Need for Respect

Every life matters. Children can teach us about this. The famous children's TV personality, Mr. Rogers, once gave a talk that included something that had happened at the Seattle Special Olympics. It goes something like this: There were nine contestants, all of them physically or mentally challenged, for the hundred-yard dash. All of them were assembled at the starting line. At the sound of the gun, they took off. Not long afterward one little boy stumbled, fell, hurt his knee, and began to cry. The other eight children heard him crying, slowed down, turned around and ran back to him. One little girl with Down syndrome bent down, kissed the boy and said, "This will make it better." The little boy got up. He and the rest of the runners linked their arms together and joyfully walked to the finish line. They all finished the race at the same time. And when they did, everyone in the stadium stood up, clapped, whistled, and cheered for a long, long time. Everybody won. If we had appropriate respect for ourselves and others, everybody would win.

Respect is indispensable. It comes from within us and sustains the ability to move forward amid confusion, distress, and contradictions. Self-respect is a sound foundation for nurturing the positive elements in our personality and our chronic disease. We must be true to ourselves. Self-respect is not for sale, and cannot be purchased, or fabricated. It is revealed to us when we are alone, in quiet moments, in quiet places, when we realize that we have done what is good, served what is beautiful, and spoken what is true.

Because they are different, people with visible physical disabilities can have low self-respect. If people have low self-respect, it is easy for them to follow the crowd, vacillate about personal preferences, be taken advantage of, or have poor decision-making skills. They can also habitually denigrate themselves or use negative self talk.

If we have a long-term serious disease, we cannot afford to be without self-respect. It is necessary for survival, especially when we are going through disturbing or downbeat times with our disease. Chronic disease brings times of crises and sober confrontation with our personal situation. To honor self-respect contributes to strength of character, keeps a disease in its right perspective, and refines what is valued. Who we are to ourselves is manifest by who we are to others. To know what is good, beautiful, and true about ourselves, will affect those around us.

Self-respect is revealed in how we interpret ourselves and the way we manage our disease. We deal with problems, honor our commitments, remain cognizant about disease concerns, and finish what we start. We realize it is not what we have, but what we do with what we have that matters.

The Essential Need for Respect

What is most important about us is invisible, like the faith, hope, and love we hold in our heart. When we are in social situations, we remain within the verbal boundaries that reinforce self-respect. For example, we refrain from talking about the woes of our disease, off-color jokes, dark conversations, or demeaning or depressing situations.

If we become stuck in a rut of negative thoughts about our disease, we can look in the mirror, smile and say out loud, "I am an honorable person." We do not let negative things other people say about our limitations influence who we are. Does anyone on this earth really know us?

A chronic condition may cause us to need extra time to do a task, experience difficulty walking, or ask someone to assist us with something we can no longer do alone. If there is something that we cannot do because of our chronic disease, we should not belabor the fact or think poorly of ourselves. Limitations from a chronic disease are not failures. It is self-defeating to attach our self-worth to a condition or event regarding our disease. Just because a person cannot do something does not mean that he or she is a dysfunctional person. It is important to love ourselves as integrated individuals. If we look at admirable public people who have, or have had, a serious disease, we admire them more because of their serious disease. If we look around, we find that people with infirmities can embrace life most admirably.

To see ourselves primarily as people of worth is an asset to navigate through a serious chronic disease. Even though it takes up time and energy, a disease is far from the only, or the most important, component of our identity. We need to ignore society's emphasis on looks, youth, and what is currently fashionable. When societal expectations come to mind, we remember that the final word regarding how we fit into society depends on us, not others. Our actions are guided by personal values, which may become more refined because of our disease. What we value is underlined by what we believe and is supported by our daily behavior and decisions. Our values affirm who we are and how we respond in social situations. It is better to displease people by doing what we know is right than to temporarily please them by doing what we know is wrong. When we value what illuminates good, beauty, and truth, we give to others a deeper understanding of life and love. This is not as hard as it may seem. Sometimes all a person needs is a hand to hold and a heart to understand.

Margaret of Castello

Margaret was born in 1287 to a noble family in the castle of Metola, which is near Florence, Italy. She was a dwarf, blind, had curvature of the spine, and difficulty walking due to a malformed short right leg. Her parents kept her out of sight because they were ashamed of her and told people she had died during childbirth. They kept her hidden in a secluded room of the castle. A kindly maid cared for Margaret. When Margaret was six, she accidentally became known to a guest, and her parents moved her to a cell attached to a church where she stayed for fourteen years. Margaret was able to talk to the priest, hear Mass, and receive communion through a window that looked into the church.

When she was twenty, her parents, seeking a miracle, took her to the tomb of a holy Franciscan named Fra Giacomo, who was buried in the Franciscan church in Citta di Castello. It was reported that miracles happened at his tomb.

The Essential Need for Respect

When no miracle occurred, they abandoned Margaret and left her in the church. Margaret's faith and courage gained the love of a few good, poor women who helped her. Later, she entered a cloistered convent. However, her sincere faith and dedication to an austere lifestyle caused the nuns, who were used to a comfortable lifestyle, to send her away. Taken in by a villager, Margaret became acquainted with a lay Dominican community, joined them, and helped them with their service to the underprivileged. She lived an exemplary life of prayer, and regularly visited and comforted the poor, the sick, and prisoners. So impressed were those whom she visited that many returned to the Church. Even though her upbringing was far from normal, she loved her parents and maintained a cheerful disposition throughout her life.

Margaret did not allow her disabilities to lead her to self-pity or bitterness. She focused on the love of God and brought that love to those around her. She saw with the eyes of spiritual wisdom. People focused on her compassion and kindness rather than on her disabilities. She never complained, lost heart, or became discouraged. Margaret looked at suffering with the eyes of faith. She did not know why God permitted her to have so many afflictions, but did know that he was an infinitely loving Father. Margaret's patience and deep faith were an inspiration to many. She died in 1330, at the age of thirty-three. A great crowd gathered for her funeral. They requested that she be buried inside the church. The priest refused. However, when a girl disabled by an accident was miraculously cured by touching Margaret's coffin, the priest relented. Margaret's life demonstrates why we need to respect and honor the dignity of all people, no matter what their challenges. Margaret of Castello is the patron saint of people with disabilities and of the pro-life movement. She was canonized on April 24, 2021.

The Importance of Self-Control

A key factor that supports self-respect is self-control, a life long task of governing body, mind, and spirit. Self-control modifies overpowering moods and feelings that accompany a chronic disease. We are neither too hard or critical, nor too soft or indulgent with ourselves. We have no control over what another person thinks about us, but we do regarding what we think. Our belief in God and subsequently in ourselves, controls losing our temper, or commonsense, amid the paradoxes of our disease. We try to transcend what is disturbing during difficult days, and enjoy days when symptoms are quiet. Self-control avoids impulsive decisions and magnifying or minimizing health care issues. Dealing with physical limits, or exacerbated symptoms, requires focused energy. Self-control as stability recognizes problems that must be addressed. When we are quiet and still, problems can clarify themselves. We face them, get help to deal with them if necessary, and make plans to resolve, or work with, them.

Self-control helps us live within the boundaries of our physical limitations. For example, a mom who has significant arthritis in her hands would like to cook dinner in a half hour like she used to do, but that is no longer realistic. Now she includes utilizing adaptive kitchen aids, conserves her energy, and budgets additional time for the tasks. She achieves the same results through altered means. She may not be able to do something one way, like opening a jar with her hands, but she can do it in another way, by using a serrated jar opener. Whatever our limitations are, we respect them along with other parts of our chronic disease. If we have a lifetime limitation, so what? No one is perfect, and every person, and task, is equal in importance.

An Easier Way through the Day

Chronic disease takes its toll in lowered energy and stamina, as well as physical limits. This makes doing many activities difficult. It gives our self-respect a boost when we do something we thought we could no longer do. There is usually more than one way to do a task and it may even turn out to be a better, easier way. Here are some suggestions to consider:

Before Tasks: Prepare a time plan. List the day of the week across the top of a page. Mark hourly segments from rising to going to bed down the left side of page.

List what you do in the appropriate time slot. For each task, ask: Why is it necessary? What is the best way of doing it? Place essential high-energy jobs at peak energy periods. Alternate active jobs and quiet jobs, standing/walking jobs and sitting jobs, heavy jobs and light jobs, jobs done with others and jobs done alone. Allow for a rest break after each high-energy job. Set realistic expectations. If a task is moderately heavy, long, or tedious, allow time for short rest breaks during the task. Eliminate steps within a task, or whole tasks, if they are not essential. Assign age-appropriate household chores to family members. When people offer to help, give them specific tasks to do.

During Tasks: Store items used often within easy reach, use vertical storage (for large, flat dishes, baking pans, griddles, cookie sheets), pull out shelves, peg boards, lazy susans.

Store items seldom used in a remote area. Before starting a task, gather necessary supplies and place in order of use. Strive to work at a slow, steady pace. Use strength from large muscle groups rather than small muscles (for example, use a shoulder strap instead of a hand held purse). Sit to do a task when possible. Limit sudden or prolonged strain, bending, multitasking, and undue anxiety. Rest before becoming exhausted. Find easier ways to do things. Ask household members to put their belongings and laundry in the proper place and to keep their rooms tidy.

Household Tips: Frozen entrees reduce food preparation. Use casserole dishes for cooking and serving. Use large dishes and pots with double handles for easier lifting. Remove hot foods with a strainer basket or slotted spoon instead of lifting the pot to drain or pour. Soak dirty dishes immediately after use. Use a wheeled utility table and objects with casters or wheels. Slide heavy objects already on the counter instead of lifting them. Use electrically powered appliances. Use light-weight dishes, pans, utensils, bowls, etc. Buy household supplies and groceries in small quantity packages. Use scissors for opening "tear here" packaged perishables, etc. Use stabilizers (suction bases, vises, lid openers, non-skid mats) to avoid holding objects in hands for long periods of time. Do a little cleaning each day, vacuum one day, dust the next, clean the bathroom the following day; or clean a room a day. Do light once-overs to avoid dirt accumulation.

Live Simply: Have a centrally located bulletin board with space for a large family appointment calendar, shopping lists, household telephone numbers, note pad for reminders and inspirational thoughts, and photographs. For emergencies:

The Essential Need for Respect

Maintain a container of large index cards, one card for each family member. On each card write the following: Name, birth date, emergency contact and phone number, current doctors and their phone numbers, current prescriptions, over the counter and herbal medications, medical conditions, allergies/sensitivities, major illnesses, chronic disorders, immunizations and surgeries. Make a copy of this information (especially medications) and keep in wallet for every doctor's visit, so that each doctor will know what medications/supplements you are taking. Know the location of advance directives. Keep medication caddie in a place where you will remember to take daily medications. Give away possessions not needed, or not used during the year. Avoid clutter on counters and in other work areas.

Self Care: Avoid long hot showers or baths. Sit to dress with all clothes needed next to you. Wear clothes that do not need ironing. Participating in a favored pastime, like playing tennis, may no longer be possible, but a new pastime, like creating ceramics, may be just as rewarding. Take short walks and do endurance and resistive exercises to tolerance. Work on mind-stimulating games like crossword puzzles, spelling games, word searches, word matches, jeopardy, sudoku. Play board games, listen to music, read, write, pray. Respect your pain, limitations and fatigue level. Live in the present, the past is history, the future is mystery. Recognize and use your talents and gifts. Be patient and gentle with yourself. Daily forgiveness keeps us from dwelling on revenge, grudges, and other destructive thoughts. Do what you can and leave the rest for another day. As far as possible be on good terms with all persons. Try to maintain a positive outlook, a sense of humor, and enjoy the lighter side of life. Reflect on the importance of faith and hope. Strive to know God, and be at peace with yourself and with the world.

Treat Your Neighbor as Yourself

A story is told about a professor who gathered his students together before the dawn. It was still very dark outside. He told them to pay attention because he had an important question to ask: How could they tell when night had ended and day had begun? One student replied: "When you see an animal and can tell whether it is a sheep or a dog?" "No," said the professor. Another student replied: "When you look at a tree in the distance and can tell whether it is a fig tree or a peach tree?" "No," answered the professor. After a few more guesses the students said, "Tell us, what is it?" The professor responded: "It is when you look into the face of any man or woman and see that he is your brother or she is your sister. If you cannot do this, no matter what time it is, it will always be night."

The measure of our self-respect is reflected in the measure of our respect for others, no matter what their race, religion, or ethnicity. Chronic disease is a common bond within the human family. It unites us when we help, and learn from each other. Although two people with the same disease experience it differently, they can support and encourage each other. Each individual is unique, and is formed beyond the influence of family, culture, or society. Growth as a human family requires effort and struggle. Conflict, pain, and sorrow can help us to grow. A certain toughness resists the many aspects of negativity in humanity, and allows us to care for others without internalizing or getting emotionally unbal-

The Essential Need for Respect

anced by their problems, or taking on their problems as our own. True caring is not a martyrdom that works us to the bone, or drives us beyond our limits. Rather, it is the willingness to accept responsibility for sustaining life, provide reasonable care for others, and do things necessary for good will and compassionate living. All persons are created equal and deserve basic human rights. Dealing with the many facets of disease reveals that every life matters, and there is more that unites than divides us.

Michelangelo could look at a plain block of marble and see within this cold, formless stone something precious. He could transform a useless chunk of marble into something beautiful because he saw what was locked inside. If we believe we are human beings created in the image and likeness of God, we know that within each of us are elements of what is good, noble, and beautiful. The artist inside us challenges us to see these elements and others within ourselves regardless of differences that separate us. We must activate and remain aware of the artist in us in order to see beyond the surface level of others.

A woman named Francoise came to a L'Arche community. She could not speak, dress herself, eat by herself, was incontinent, and walked with much difficulty. She was at the community for thirty years and became blind. At that time a visitor saw Francoise and asked the leader what was the point of keeping her alive? She only saw Francoise as someone who needed much care. The leader of the house loved Francoise for who she was. He saw her as a unique individual, with strengths and weaknesses like himself. The visitor did not realize Francoise had inner beauty which was the focus of the house leader. The presence of a chronic disease or a disability does not define a person's quality of life or level of happiness.

In his book *The Moral Sense*, James Q. Wilson wrote, "Mankind's moral sense is not a strong beacon light, radiating outward to illuminate in sharp outline all that it touches. It is, rather, a small candle flame, casting vague and multiple shadows, flickering and sputtering in the strong winds of power and passion, greed and ideology. But brought close to the heart and cupped in one's hands, it dispels the darkness and warms the soul."[1] Those of us with chronic diseases should be those small candle flames.

That small candle flame is precious and we need to safeguard it and keep it close to our heart, for it serves as the morning star on our moral compass. It represents who we are at our inmost center, what we honor, and is the wellspring of our being. Moral strength fortifies self-respect by validating how we wish to be treated and what we expect from others in terms of dignity. Our flame must remain strong to give light to others through our good example. A strong flame is sustained by striving to be honest, diligent, polite, obeying authority, honoring promises, cooperating with others, assisting those in need, and living out our religious beliefs. Our chronic disease can slow us down. However, in our slowness, we can ruminate on the importance of these qualities.

In a speech he made to the young people of South Africa, at the University of Cape Town on their Day of Affirmation in 1966, Robert F. Kennedy said, "Few will have the greatness to bend history itself, but each of us can work to change a small portion of events, and in the total of all those acts will be written the history of this generation. It is from number-

The Essential Need for Respect

less diverse acts of courage and belief that human history is shaped. Each time a man stands up for an ideal, or acts to improve the lot of others, or strikes out against injustice, he sends forth a tiny ripple of hope, and crossing each other from a million different centers of energy and daring, those ripples build a current that can sweep down the mightiest walls of oppression and resistance."[2] How are we a ripple of hope?

Wisdom through the Ages

Spiritual practices sustain and strengthen discerning what is true and right in decisions or actions about our chronic disease. These practices bond us with God. The foundation for self-respect is that God knows all about us and loves us unconditionally. In Isaiah 43:4 God said, "Because you are precious in my eyes, and honored, and I love you." He created each person in a loving and special way. If we strive to see ourselves as God sees us, we realize that there are things about us unknown to us. However, they are known by God and may be revealed to us in the future. He sees good things in us that we do not see. Like seeds in the ground, at the right time and with the right nourishment we will bloom.

Francis was born into a wealthy family in Italy. During his youth he enjoyed parties, had many friends, was charming and affable, wore fancy clothes and was quite fond of good times. He spent money freely indulging his whims and enjoyed serenading pretty girls. People saw that he was popular, suave, debonair and fun-loving, but God saw much more. When he was in his early twenties, Frances laid aside his worldly pleasures and took up a life of poverty dedicating himself to God. He became known as God's troubadour and attracted many followers who radically lived the teachings of the Gospel in a fresh and far reaching way. "Francis' health was almost certainly compromised from his early adulthood, and continued to worsen throughout his life until, on the eve of his death, he was so infirm he could not walk, was suffering from unspecified illnesses of the spleen, liver and stomach, and had a significant visual impairment."[3] Today, Francis of Assisi has an almost universal appeal. He is the best known of the saints and attracts people who are interested in ecology, peace, gardening, animals, a simple life style, joyful singing, and living like Jesus. On his feast day, October 4th, even unbelievers come to parish parking lots to get their pets blessed.

Prayer helps us to maintain respect for ourselves and others. There are hundreds of gates into a prayer garden, and we must find our own gate. One gate opens into silence, a treasure for prayer. Distracting noises are stilled outside so we can hear more easily the soft quiet voice of God deep within us. We need time to be alone and silent, to reflect and to listen his voice. Prayer keeps us humble. Humility helps us to respect all people as equal members of God's family.

There is a story—I do not know its source—about an old man and a young man on the same platform before a huge audience. A special program was being presented. As part of this program, each man was to repeat from memory the words of the Twenty-Third Psalm. The young man trained in the best speech technique and drama, gave, in the language of an ancient silver-tongued orator, the words of the psalm. "The Lord is my shepherd . . . ." When he had finished, the audience clapped their hands and cheered, asking him for

The Essential Need for Respect

an encore so that they might hear again his wonderful voice. Then the old gentleman, leaning heavily on his cane, stepped to the front of the same platform, and in feeble, shaking voice, repeated the same words—"The Lord is my shepherd … " But when he was seated no sound came from the listeners. Folks seemed to pray. In the silence the young man stood to make the following statement: "Friends," he said. "I wish to make an explanation. You asked me to come back and repeat the psalm, but you remained silent when my friend here was seated. The difference? I shall tell you. I know the psalm, but he knows the shepherd."[4]

When Jesus, the Good Shepherd, knocks at our door, may we never be too preoccupied to hear him. Silence offers an environment for serious thought that leads to action in the marketplace. When World War II ended, a young American soldier came upon a Catholic church in a small French town. A statue of Jesus was lying on the ground. He picked it up and saw that it was intact, except the hands of Jesus were broken off. The soldier took some paper from his bag, wrote a message, and placed the paper at the base of the statue. The message he wrote was: I have no hands but yours. Indeed, words to ponder.

Folding our hands in prayer for those who are hurting within the human family is most valuable. How many people don't have anyone to pray for them? Prayer for others is a service of the heart, and helps us to bear our own suffering with patience and hope. We accept what we cannot do because of our chronic disease and strive to walk in the footsteps of Jesus. We look calmly at our crucifix and go beyond emotion. Gazing at the crucifix uncovers the extraordinary treasure of strength and courage in trials. This discovery destroys bitterness and distrust in us, which makes us peaceful people. Jesus' crucifixion shows that the more love an individual brings into a situation the more vulnerable she becomes. Loving makes us vulnerable, but even so, love has triumphed over hate. On the cross Jesus made known that evil was mastered by good and hate was overcome by love.

When we experience common struggles, we can come together for support and encouragement. This can provide a level of healing and help that goes beyond that of health care professionals. Our faith decreases our fears and doubts, enables us to go forward with greater trust and confidence in God, and sustains a renewed vision of life. Hope keeps us from discouragement and sustains our belief in Divine Providence. Love is the most brilliant jewel in the crown of virtues because it animates and inspires the practice of all virtues. We need love to release us from being bogged down by disease-related concerns. In those concerns, we can find a hidden gift, or message of God's love, if we look for it. Trials can teach us truths, about God, or about parts of ourselves we do not like and have buried deep inside us. Living day after day with a chronic disease can lead to conversion toward God, and blessings that come from limitations. This can happen when people who have left their religion for one reason or another, return to it. They see and understand things that they did not see or understand before.

Love opens us to greater wonder. No guide will tell us what will happen on the road ahead, but love enlightens us to rare beauty, thoughtful listening, and deep thinking. Love is the supreme gift from heaven, and the greatest good on earth.

The Essential Need for Respect

We could not manage our chronic disease without signs of God's love around us. In 1861, Horatius Bonar wrote this beautiful hymn, "O Love of God, How Strong and True."

> O love of God, how strong and true!
> Eternal and yet ever new;
> Uncomprehended and unbought,
> Beyond all knowledge and all thought.
>
> O love of God, how deep and great!
> Far deeper than man's deepest hate;
> Self-fed, self-kindled, like the light,
> Changeless, eternal, infinite.
>
> O heav'nly love, how precious still,
> In days of weariness and ill!
> In nights of pain and helplessness,
> To heal, to comfort, and to bless.
>
> O wide embracing, wondrous love,
> We read Thee in the sky above,
> We read Thee in the earth below,
> In seas that swell, and streams that flow.
>
> We read Thee in the flowers, the trees,
> The freshness of the fragrant breeze,
> The song of birds upon the wing,
> The joy of summer and of spring.
>
> We read Thee best in Him who came
> To bear for us the cross of shame;
> Sent by the Father from on high,
> Our life to live, our death to die.

Courage through Chronic Disease

We read Thee in the manger-bed,
On which His infancy was laid;
And Nazareth that love reveals,
Nestling amid its lonely hills.

We read Thee in the tears once shed,
Over doomed Salem's guilty head,
In the cold tomb of Bethany,
And blood-drops of Gethsemane.

We read Thy power to bless and save,
E'en in the darkness of the grave;
Still more in resurrection light,
We read the fullness of Thy might.

O love of God, our shield and stay
Through all the perils of our way;
Eternal love, in Thee we rest,
Forever safe, forever blest!

Notes

1. James Q. Wilson, *The Moral Sense* (New York, NY: Free Press Paperbacks, 1993), 251.
2. Edward Kennedy, "Eulogy of Robert F. Kennedy," New York, NY, June 8, 1968, http://www.speeches-usa.com/Transcripts/ted_kennedy-eulogyofRFK.html.
3. Donna Trembinski, *Before a Saint, A Man: Disability in the Life of Francis of Assisi,* November 20, 2020, https://utorontopress.com/blog/2020/11/20/trembinski-disability-in-the-life-of-francis-of-assisi/.
4. Charles L. Allen, *God's Psychiatry* (Westwood, NJ: Fleming H. Revell Company, 1953), 38.

Chapter 11

Finding Harmony

A physical disability can result from a disease, injury, accident or be present at birth. Dominican Brother Vincent, of the Irish Dominican province, is a splendid example of how a person with a physical disability can foster harmony and goodness in those with whom he lives and works. Father Timothy Radcliffe writes:

> Vincent was blind from birth. He never saw another human face. He entered the Order when he was young and soon became one of the most beloved members of the province. This is partly because he was a deeply lovable person, who was strong and humorous, and had utterly no self-pity.
> When I was provincial every community asked me if I would assign Vincent to their community. Not only was it because he was loveable, Vincent gathered community around him. You cannot have someone in the community who is totally blind unless you really are a community. You have to ensure that nothing is in his way when he feels his way down the corridors, and that the milk in the fridge is always in exactly the same place, so that he can find it. All our decisions about our com-

mon life had to have Vincent in mind. And this is not a burden but a joy, since around him we discover each other. He summons us beyond the silly Western illusion that anyone is self-sufficient. In his needs, we discover our own need for each other. He frees us to be brothers, mutually dependent.

Because he was blind, he depended upon his hearing. He heard sound bounce off the walls. He navigated around the rooms with his ears. And this meant that he was wonderfully sensitive to what the brethren say. He was appointed to the Formation Team, because he could spot what was happening in the lives of the young, their strengths and weaknesses, more than most of us. His disability was a gift. He picked up the nuances that others miss. He heard our secret fears and hopes in our voices. We are all blind and deaf in some way, and sometimes the blind teach us to hear and the deaf teach us to see, and the lame give us the courage to take another step.[1]

In 1971 there was a happy TV commercial that became a popular song. The first line was: "I'd like to teach the world to sing in perfect harmony." This is a heart-warming concept ever waiting to become a reality. Many people understood that "sing" was actually a metaphor for "live." Living in harmony with others is a most beautiful endeavor and an ongoing challenge. However, harmony begins from within, when what we believe, think, say, and do are in agreement.

We will slip into pessimism at times, perhaps many times, during the duration of our disease. This is normal but we must not stay there. We try to maintain an optimistic attitude. What can we do to decrease pessimistic thinking?

Finding Harmony

We express feelings about our serious disease by saying we are discouraged or apathetic. Then we remember something good, like someone's love for us, or a fine meal. When we feel flattened by the frustrations of a chronic disease, we can find help by the first three steps of the twelve-step program of Alcoholics Anonymous: (1) admit we are powerless in this area; (2) believe in the higher power of God to help us; (3) and decide to turn this weakness, and our entire lives, over to God. These steps fortify hope for the best, especially when our disease has really got us down. We can counteract a dissonant thought by replacing it with a calming thought, write down disturbing ruminations and then burn the paper in the fireplace, challenge a troubling assumption with the facts, disperse the gloom by recalling a pleasant experience or listening to a favorite old song. We can assertively say "Stop!" to downward spiral thoughts. As Augustine said regarding temptations and unwanted thoughts, they can fly around our heads but they need not make a nest in our hair. Pessimistic thoughts can make us our own worst enemy. It is much better to be our own best friend.

    Praying to God, who is far beyond yet deep within us, can elevate our thoughts. This short prayer has given many people courage to go on: "Jesus, I give my life to you." When we say yes to God's graces, depression morphs into hope, deflation to engagement, and withdrawal to commitment. Welcoming grace confirms there is more good in life than what is perceived through feelings and the senses. Religious tenets and practices can be enormous supports on a harmonic life-long journey. We are bearers of God's love by living a steadfast Christian way of life and through it promoting dignity of human life.

We Are Not Alone

Gerhard Frost wrote: "'The reason mountain climbers are tied together is to keep the sane ones from going home.' I don't know who said it, or when or where, but I've chuckled over it, thought about it, and quoted it, too. With a mountain of mercy behind me and a mountain of mission ahead, I need you, my sister, my brother; I need to be tied to you, and you need me, too. We need each other . . . to keep from bolting, fleeing in panic, and returning to the 'sanity' of unbelief. Wise words, whoever said them; I've placed them in my Bible."[2] We need each other to work toward harmony. Survival means staying connected because every person counts.

Harmony develops by using freedom the right way. We are free to the extent that we do not limit another person's freedom. A common example is playing music so loud that it disturbs others. The choice to blast one's music is made without concern about how it will affect others who are nearby. This choice disrupts peaceful, harmonic living. We cannot do what we want to do when we want to do it. Yes, we are free to choose the volume of our music, but we must consider others when doing so. If harmony is a priority, it shifts our focus from self-interests to the common good. In the long run, doing things for others is more rewarding than doing things for ourselves.

A long term disease can inspire ideas that lead to constructive change. We can improve adaptive devices, like a sock cone or dressing stick (tools to help us dress from socks to

Finding Harmony

shirt). Our idea can be original in its adaptation to the problem on which we are working. And there are several problems we would not have if we did not have a chronic disease. How could our solutions help others, especially those with the same disease as ours?

Harmony blossoms when people care for each other. The famed anthropologist Margaret Mead was once asked what she considered to be the earliest sign of civilization. She responded that it was a human femur (thigh bone) with a healed fracture. One had been excavated from a fifteen-thousand-year-old site. For a human being to have survived a broken femur, he would have required shelter, food, drink, and protection throughout the months it took for the femur to heal. Clearly this early human was a recipient of care and attention from fellow humans. Compassion leads us to avoid being indifferent to the suffering of others. Regardless of age, profession, health, education, or wealth, we must discover a path to living together cooperatively and working together for the betterment of all. We share blessings and burdens, defending what is right and confronting what is wrong to clear up indignities to human life.

A basic loyalty to a person who has physical restrictions means watching, waiting, keeping company with and standing by him or her in times of pain or anguish. Loyalty is not dependent on words, but an unexplainable form of compassion. Everyone needs help of some kind. Helping to carry another's burdens is a sign of our common humanity. Quality of life is based more on who we are in the light of God's love, and less on productivity, outward appearance, or successes.

Putting Labels on People

When we draw our own conclusions about who is weak and who is strong, our perceptions are wanting. The value of human life should be based on respect for the equality of human beings, not their differences. We concentrate on what we have in common. Negative labels can tear harmony to shreds. Normal and abnormal are labels. Like good and bad, sick and well, normal is considered beautiful, acceptable, and positive, and abnormal is considered unsightly, unwanted, and negative. Whether positive or negative, labeling people is risky. It can lead to mind sets, affirm negative mental images, support inaccurate attitudes, and over simplify situations. Labels lead to attitudinal barriers. A person who has a physical handicap that is a result of a disease or injury may feel less limited by the handicap than by the attitudes of others regarding the handicap.

Person-first language puts the person before his or her disease or disability. Isn't it more respectful to say the man who is blind, rather than the blind man? Adults with physical disabilities must be treated as adults. Guidelines for "normal" people are: They must not, literally or figuratively, talk down to those who are physically limited, speak as if they were children, or make decisions they can make themselves. They speak directly to a person with a disability, not to his or her companion. They do not assume what he or she needs, but asks if they want assistance. They should not touch or move mobility equipment such as a wheelchair, scooter, walker or cane without permission, because they are extensions of a person. People without physical limits should never make fun of a person with a disability, mimic, or act as if they have one. Because of our fallen humanity, isn't everyone disabled in some way? Physical disability is an overemphasized term, and stigmatized by negative assumptions and discrimination. A disability is only one component of an individual. It can happen to anyone at anytime and should not be a reason for inequity or stereotypes.

Jean Vanier, the founder of L'Arche, taught us much about the value of a suffering person's life. He believed that imperfections and fallibilities are important but overlooked aspects of being human. Shared fragility has the potential to unite us. People can thrive, and become closer, when they are welcomed with their gifts and their weaknesses. The weak can help the strong to accept and integrate their own weaknesses and brokenness. Jean saw how sharing weakness and difficulties were more beneficial to others than sharing qualities and successes.

To speak and listen to others in a way that reveals their beauty, worth, and importance is to see reality through the eyes of others, and be moved by their wounds. Showing a genuine interest in a person should precede doing things for him or her. We think about what it would be like to be in their place. When we begin to authentically listen to each other's stories, we move from exclusion to inclusion, from fear to trust, from being closed to being open, and from judgment to forgiveness. Such are movements of the heart. They do not mean doing great or extraordinary things, but doing ordinary things with sensitivity, gentleness, and forgiveness. If we love people as they are with their wounds and their gifts, rather than how we want them to be, we create harmony. Sharing our weaknesses and difficulties without being self-absorbed can create a strong bond among people.

In his elder years, during an interview, Jean gave good advice for inner harmony. He said he had his weaknesses, fragility, and physical ailments of the heart. He had to take things quietly. Intellectually, he got tired much more quickly. He had a greater need for sleep and took a nap after lunch. This was his present reality which he accepted. He advises us to live the reality of today and not live in the imagination, in what could have been, what should have been or, we can add, what might be in the future, because we do not know what our future on earth will bring. Whatever our future brings, we are all moving toward the ultimate reality which is death. We need not be frightened of death. It is a passage of extraordinary discovery. A rebirth that will be so amazing that we cannot even imagine it.

Patience and flexibility are necessary to cope with the concerns of the moment. Daily living in community provides plenty of ways to practice compassion. Therese of Lisieux gives us a practical example. When she was in the convent, she helped an old, crotchety nun to walk along the corridors. Therese received a continuum of complaints: "You move too fast." Therese slowed down. "Well, come on, now you are too slow." Therese walked a bit faster. "I don't feel your hand, you let go of me and I'm going to fall." Therese tightened her grasp. "I was right when I said you were too young to help me." Therese smiled. Even though the sister's complaints seemed endless, Therese took it all in stride, and did not let it bother her. The sister's grumbles did not disturb Therese because she saw beyond them which helped her respond with

Finding Harmony

a tender heart and patient demeanor. Therese learned to love the cranky dear old nun through a compassionate act that created harmony.[3]

The blessings of harmony that lie beneath the turbulence of a chronic disease take time to surface. Harmony is not a matter of intensity but of balance, order, rhythm, and unity. It is reinforced by an innate need to connect with and value that which is enduring, tried and tested. How can we appreciate what is deep within us during the storms of a chronic disease? Living with chronic infirmities can slow us down and give us the time to reflect and ponder. This may compel us to collect and safeguard stories that ensure lessons in our personal history are not lost. These histories may include family, religion, school, community, country, or endearing organizations to which we belonged. Stories connect us with the past and give stability to the present. Living with a serious disease can encourage us to become mentors or teachers to others through stories about our own grief, joy, struggles, successes, and faith. When we retell our stories we can gain, and record, new insights and interpretations. We may smile with gratitude when our experience of chronic disease helps others. Everyone with a serious disease has their own unique story to tell.

We cannot grow without knowing from where we came. We need to keep significant memories alive, both the good and the bad, so we can celebrate the good and try not to repeat the bad. Even though our bodies change, the essence of who we are can strengthen and sustain us. A stable sense of personal history reveals future possibilities that are examined by the heart and the head. Long-term disease can initiate the deepening, softening, healing, and strengthening of our personal characteristics.

Better Safe than Sorry

Safety first changes from a proverb to a lived reality. Prevention is easier than a cure.

If we are physically compromised by an unstable gate, balance problems, sensory loss, or muscle weakness, we must adhere to safety rules because painful bruises, broken bones or worse, from sudden disharmonious events are not welcome. Because falling is a major fear, here are a few suggestions with an invitation to add to them as they come to mind:

Keep muscles as strong as possible. Wear properly fitting, flat, sturdy shoes with nonskid soles. Hold on to sturdy handrails when going up or down steps or stairs (inside and outside). Carefully go up, or down, steps one at a time or use a chair lift.

When walking outside, without help, or with a walker or cane, watch for uneven sidewalks and lift up your feet. At home, keep walkways and room floors clear of clutter, including cables or other cords. Remove loose rugs. Use non-slip treads on bare-wood steps. If there is need to hold on to furniture when walking, make sure the furniture is sturdy. At night, keep night lights on in bedroom, bathroom, and hallways. When in bed, be sure a phone and flashlight are within reach. Organize items used everyday so that their height is between your shoulders and waist. Use long-handled reachers to pick things up from the floor but do not try to get items from overhead. If something is out of reach, use a sturdy step ladder and not a chair. Use chairs with arm rests and high-rise pillow. Use non-slip mats or decals and grab bars in bathtub or shower. Use a bath seat with hand-held shower nozzle. Use a raised toilet seat with arm rests.

Do not delay: If there is a spill, wipe it up. If it is empty, fill it. If it is moved, put it back. If it is open, close it. If it is broken, fix it. If it is used up, put it on the shopping list. If you fall, and you are by yourself, have a plan regarding how you are going to get up or who you are going to call.

The Circle of Life

Endings connect with beginnings. Spring follows winter, dawn follows darkness, and each individual comes from God, lives, dies, and returns to God. Beginnings and endings are like a circle. In the great circle of life, just as each member of a family is part of the family circle, so each nation is a part of the world. There is no first or last, superior or inferior, better or worse. Harmony is what all humanity needs; a way of life with origins in a love that sees each person as a neighbor. The vicissitudes of frail health can teach us to be loving and patient toward ourselves and others. The power of harmony infuses calm and quiet that helps to endure our disease. Love is the most necessary component of harmony and asks for more than seems possible. Genuine love rouses us out of mediocrity, and requires work, effort, and sacrifice.

In the fifteenth century, in a tiny village near Nuremberg, there lived a family with eighteen children. In order to feed his family, the father, a goldsmith, worked almost eighteen hours a day at his trade and at any other job he could find. Despite their meager existence, two of the children had a dream. They both wanted to pursue the study of art. However, they knew their father would not be financially able to send either of them to Nuremberg to study at the academy.

Courage through Chronic Disease

After long discussions the two boys worked out a pact. They would toss a coin. The loser would work in the nearby mines and his earnings would support his brother who would attend the academy. Then, when that brother finished his studies, he would support the other brother as he attended the academy. They tossed a coin after church one Sunday. Albrecht Durer won the toss and went off to Nuremberg. His brother, Albert, went off to the mines and worked in them for four years. As was promised, he financed his brother, whose work at the academy was quite a sensation. Albrecht's etchings, woodcuts, and oils were better than those of many of his professors.

When the young artist returned to his village, the Durer family held a festive dinner to celebrate. After a memorable meal, Albrecht rose from his place of honor and made a toast to his beloved brother. At the end he told Albert that it was his turn. He could go to Nuremberg to pursue his dream and Albrecht would take care of him. Albert shook his lowered head. He said no, he could not go to Nuremberg. It was too late. Four years in the mines destroyed his hands. The bones in his fingers were often broken because of his work. His hands were stiff and sore. The arthritis was so bad in his right hand that he could not hold a glass to return the toast. To draw delicate lines on canvas would be impossible.

More than 450 years have passed. Albrecht Durer's masterful portraits, woodcuts, sketches, and other works are in great museums all over the world. However, more people are probably familiar with only one of his works. One day, to pay homage to Albert for all he had sacrificed, Albrecht painstakingly drew his brother's bruised hands with palms together and fingers skyward. He called this masterpiece *Hands*. We know this tribute of love as *The Praying Hands*.

Notes

    1. Timothy Radcliffe, "A Spirituality of Suffering and Healing," *Religious Life Review* (September–October 2012).

    2. Gerhard E. Frost, "Blessed Is the Ordinary," as quoted in Charles Swindoll, *The Tale of the Tardy Oxcart and 1,501 Other Stories* (Nashville, TN: Word Pub., 1998), 597.

    3. For Therese's original story, see Marc Foley, *Story of a Soul: The Autobiography of St. Thérèse of Lisieux*, study, Kindle edition, (Washington, DC: ICS Publications, 2005), 390.

Chapter 12

The Spiritual Dimension

We often hear, "Never give up!" This quote holds true for every area in our lives, especially concerning our physical dimension, but most importantly, in our spiritual dimension.

Fr. Patrick Rager lived these words. Affectionately known as Father Paddy, he loved everything Irish, and was a man of many talents. Born on August 14, 1959, in West Homestead, Pennsylvania, he attended St. Mary Magdalene School where he volunteered as an altar server. At Central Catholic High School in Pittsburgh, Paddy excelled in both athletics and academics. Today his picture hangs in their alumni hall of fame. In 1981, he earned a bachelor's degree from Duquesne University where he studied theology and psychology. While attending Duquesne, he earned his emergency medical technician certificate and served in the Air Force Reserves for two years, achieving the rank of lieutenant. In the same year, he earned a master's degree in theology from Christ the King Seminary in New York and a master's degree in clinical psychopathology from St. Bonaventure University in New York. On May 11, 1985, he was ordained to the priesthood by

Bishop Anthony Bevilacqua at St. Paul Cathedral in Pittsburgh. His first assignment was as parochial vicar at St. Sylvester parish in Brentwood, a Pittsburgh suburb, where he served from 1985 to 1987.

The first sign of illness appeared when he was a seminarian. His knee gave out during a baseball game. More falls and weakening led to many medical tests and several misdiagnoses. Finally, after fifteen years, he received a diagnosis of ALS (amyotrophic lateral sclerosis), a slow and fatal paralysis, more commonly known as Lou Gehrig's disease.

Father Paddy's condition deteriorated and in 1987, he moved into an apartment in his parents' home. His priesthood changed direction there. Although he was confined to a wheelchair and eventually bedridden, he did not stop serving others. He wrote articles for Catholic publications. He developed a telephone and mail ministry that offered prayer, support, encouragement, and counseling for persons with disabilities. After an article about him appeared in a national Catholic newsweekly, this ministry expanded to people in different areas of the world. Even with his many physical limitations, Father Paddy's priesthood was incredibly alive and strong. His great love for Jesus showed in Father Paddy's joyful attitude. He would flash a radiant smile and his dark eyes lit up when a joke or funny story was afoot. He enjoyed watching football games on TV, especially when his favorite team, the Pittsburgh Steelers, played. He focused on the lighter side of things, the goodness of life, and rarely complained. He was more concerned about hearing what others had to say than talking about himself.

His strong devotion to Mary was revealed in his attentiveness and readiness to offer hope. He reminds us that

The Spiritual Dimension

storms arrive in our lives with some regularity. Many times, they arrive without warning and test our strength and resolve. In difficult circumstances, we must remember that Jesus is in the boat with us just as he was in the boat with the apostles, calming them as he rebuked the winds and the waters. For the moment, Jesus may appear silent, but he never forsakes us. When Father Paddy could no longer speak, he wrote using eye movements and a computer screen. Father Paddy's priesthood was used in a way he could not have imagined at ordination. On the 20th of July, 2010, at the age of fifty, he went home to Jesus from the home where he was born and raised.

Indeed, Father Paddy never gave up and was an example of heroic virtue. He exemplified everyday holiness in prayer, in service, and in suffering. Along with Paul the apostle, he could write: "Now I rejoice in my sufferings for your sake, and in my flesh I complete what is lacking in Christ's afflictions for the sake of his body, that is, the church" (Col. 1:24).

Today the word spirituality has many meanings. In this book it refers to our relationship with God. Is he our dear friend or a distant acquaintance? Although many of us may not be aware of it, each of us has a spiritual dimension where we perceive and communicate with God. It is the most adventuresome trajectory that takes us out of ourselves and our disease concerns, and into God and the supernatural. It reveals that we are worth more than how this world defines us. Faith in God, and practicing what we believe, provides energy to rise in the morning and fuels hope throughout the day, regardless of our physical restrictions. A vibrant spiritual dimension keeps us conscious of God, thereby giving a deeper meaning to our disease. We are rooted in faith and nurtured through worship, prayer, sacraments, rites, art, music, and other expressions that bring us closer to God and more accepting of what we cannot do.

> It was a crisp, cold day; there was plenty of ice underfoot and decorating the hedges and walks. The blue sky was cloudless and there was a brilliant sun. I looked across the landscape and found that I couldn't see everything clearly; in some places a white mist was shrouding the houses and trees. Rather than this being a disappointment, somehow it was an enhancement. The view was even more beautiful than when I have seen it before; the mist lent it a serenity and peacefulness. And I realized that for me, at least, faith is like this. In an inexplicable way, mystery actually enhances beauty and there is no need to struggle to understand everything: the Trinity, the last coming, even the problem of evil. All these are best left unfathomable. Just as the mist magically made our surroundings that morning more beautiful, so the mystery of our God reveals him to be at once more believable and more wonderful.[1]

The Deepest Mystery

It is singularly beautiful to have something beyond ourselves for which to strive. The spiritual dimension is our most precious area of development, because it animates authentic living. It is known that people with a strong religious faith have a higher level of life satisfaction, greater happiness, and lower negative consequences when faced with painful circumstances. The spiritual journey can be rich, mysterious, obscure, utterly fascinating, and radically amazing. Nothing else on earth is like it because God is beyond any human being's imagination or intelligence. As God's people, we acknowledge that he is

The Spiritual Dimension

the source for truth, beauty, goodness, unity, wisdom, love, and mystery. We ponder these attributes, are grateful for virtues that come from our disease, such as patience and tenacity, and maintain a deeper awareness of divine grace.

Grace is a mysterious reality that, if we say yes to it, increases God's life and love within us. His presence becomes more prominent. The wrappings of grace can be beautiful, ugly, familiar, or strange. Whatever the wrap, God's grace will get us through difficulties. We are receptive to the grace of God when we look beyond disease negatives and see with the positive vision of God. God uses everything, including disease, to bring about a greater good than simply human physical health and survival. Pope Benedict XVI spoke of this:

> And only when God is seen does life truly begin. Only when we meet the loving God in Christ do we know what life is. We're not some casual and meaningless product of evolution. Each of us is the result of a thought of God. Each of us is willed, each of us is loved, each of us is necessary. There is nothing more beautiful than to be surprised by the Gospel, by the encounter with Christ. There is nothing more beautiful than to know him and to speak to others of our relationship with him.[2]

Deep faith reveals certitude and mystery. Isn't this also true concerning the effects of our chronic disease? Like faith, we know and we do not know. We think we are in remission and then exacerbate, expect a good report, and it is not so good. We take medication and it does not work. God's truths can only be understood in ever deepening layers through analogues, parables, metaphors and allegories, but are never understood completely. Why a physical disease happens to us can be beyond medical explanation. Paul the apostle says what we see now is like looking through a glass darkly. Psalm 46:10 says, "Be still and know that I am God." And in awesome silent stillness, we listen.

In John 21:18, Jesus tells Peter, "Truly, truly, I say to you, when you were young, you girded yourself and walked where you would; but when you are old, you will stretch out your hands, and another will gird you and carry you where you do not wish to go." We who have a serious chronic disease can relate to these words. At any age, serious disease can take us to places where we would rather not go. It turns us around and changes our priorities. We seek qualified people to explain what is going on, and the answers may be unknown. We put pride in our pocket and ask for help. To let others help us gives us a glimpse of the goodness of God who works through them. It sheds light on a truth of life: We need God and others to help us with our problems and struggles.

Long-term disease can bring many surprises. It can open doors previously unaware to us, especially the door to the spiritual realm that can shine around and in us. Moving into it broadens our previously limited notion of who God is and what he desires from us. We can experience spiritual awakenings at any time, age, or change in our physical condition. Be it instant or incremental, chronic disease can open us to God in surprising ways. At an awakening we believe he has spoken to us or we experience an internal reality that he exists.

Our contact with others can be steps toward God: A pastor, with help from his walker, manages his parish well. A fellow patient who is near death, radiates joy. A deacon preaches a heart-moving homily from his wheelchair. Before an operation, a surgeon says, "We will take good care of you." An

The Spiritual Dimension

occupational therapist, who has multiple sclerosis, demonstrates an easier way to dress. Somehow we are transformed as the reality of God becomes factual to us. Viktor Frankl, author of the classic *Man's Search for Meaning*, found God in a Nazi concentration camp. He would look up into the sky and see beauty that the Nazis could not destroy or take from him. God can bring out what is real in the midst of suffering, John Paul II wrote, "It is suffering, more than anything else, which clears the way for the grace which transforms human souls."[3]

Our spiritual dimension does not exist above or alongside the other dimensions in our lives. It is located deep within us, below the surface concerns of our disease, and can be envisioned as a tranquil environment where the spirit of God dwells. We embark on an unending exploration that strengthens our union with God, helps us to cope with our disease, influences all aspects and activities in our life, and reaches its fullest glory beyond death. Moving forward takes us from a known, familiar landscape to an unknown, endless terrain, from comfort and complacency to an unceasing search and desire that cannot be fully satisfied. As we move ahead, our disease changes from an enemy to a teacher through greater knowledge and a new focus on God. Our degenerative disease bonds us with Jesus' suffering. At the end of Jesus' life, the worst possible thing happened to the best possible person. Nevertheless, he was also God, and his death and resurrection opened the gate of heaven to all of us. However, it is up to us to walk through that gate by preparing for it here on earth.

Physical difficulties may impair our mobility but spiritually we can soar. What are some indications that show we are growing strong spiritually? We meet our basic needs such as prayer, sleep, nutrition, and hydration. We respect what we are unable to do. We are true to God and develop personal integrity that includes disease adjustments. In sickness and in health we strive for holiness and see it in others. We hold on to the tenets of our religion through thick and thin. We learn and grow from negative experiences, and set boundaries regarding acceptable behavior. Guided by God's love for us, our daily choices reflect what we value.

Confidence in God

If we stay on the spiritual path, the journey resembles an upward spiral. Grace softens movements around complicated disease curves. We should never underestimate God's activity in us when we experience difficult times. Steady confidence in God can be likened to an airline pilot flying at night or through a storm. He depends upon radar contact with the control tower to keep on course. The pilot is able to arrive at the destination without seeing the way ahead. We make our way through disease darkness and trials by using prayer as a radar of sorts. There are times when we feel we are going off course, or cannot see what lies ahead, but if we maintain contact with God, we will arrive at the destination intended for us. We keep moving in darkness and storms because we truly believe God is in control.

God's strength and grace are sturdy assets in managing our disease. Grace helps us to remove, or deal with, doubts and uncertainties. When we feel defeated or desolate, or experience a faltering faith, yet truly trust in God, we move to higher ground and see the terrain around us more clearly. God uses us in ways never imagined if we did not have our disease. Confidence in God imparts courage to move beyond negative or ambivalent feelings or hesitation. Asking for God's help is not a sign of weakness, but rather confirms our reliance on him and refines us. If we think we are lacking confidence in God, we tell him and trust him in our weakness. God does not mind hearing this. Choosing to trust him in spite of what we physically fear is truly living our faith.

A sick man turned to his doctor as he was preparing to leave the examination room and said, "Doctor, I am afraid to die. Tell me what lies on the other side." Very quietly, the doctor said, "I don't know." "You don't know? You, a Christian man, do not know what is on the other side?" The doctor was holding the handle of the door. On the other side came a sound of scratching and whining and as he opened the door, a dog sprang into the room and leaped on him with an eager show of gladness. Turning to the patient, the doctor said, "Did you notice my dog? He's never been in this room before. He didn't know what was inside. He knew nothing except that his master was here and when the door opened, he sprang in without fear. I know little of what is on the other side of death, but I do know one thing. I know my Master is there and that is enough."

Deserts of the Soul

We cannot journey through the spiritual dimension without passing through deserts that are often dry, empty, and seemingly trackless with unseen prickly cactuses that stick us when we least expect it. We do not know where we are going or what will happen. Thomas Merton prayed:

> My Lord God, I have no idea where I am going. I do not see the road ahead of me. I cannot know for certain where it will end. Nor do I really know myself, and the fact that I think I am following your will does not mean that I am actually doing so. But I believe that the desire to please you does in fact please you. And I hope I have that desire in all that I am doing. I hope I will never do anything apart from that desire. And I know that if I do you will lead me by the right road, though I may know nothing about it. Therefore I will trust you always though I may seem to be lost and in the shadow of death. I will not fear, for you are ever with me, and you will never leave me to face my perils alone.[4]

The desert trail can cause us to run away in fear and trembling or to move forward in mystery and trust. We learn how to trust and hope in God for his own sake, rather than for the things he can give us. We may see spiritual things that were not perceivable before our disease. Accepting suffering is a process that can bring our heart, mind, and soul closer to God. When we are in great pain, prayer is simple and direct. We ask God for strength to hold on. Like fire that refines gold, suffering refines us by increasing inner strength, endurance, and resiliency. We cannot know who we really are until we are tested. However, an inner calm assures us of God's protection despite physical hardships and turmoil.

Rev. John F. Chaplain wrote the following meditation.

> In pastures green? Not always. Sometimes. He who knoweth best, in kindness leadeth me in weary ways,

where heavy shadows be. Out of the sunshine warm and soft and bright, out of the sunshine into darkest night, I oft would faint with sorrow and affright. Only for this. I know he holds my hand, so whether led in the green or desert land, I trust, although I may not understand. And by still waters? No, not always so, often times the heavy tempests round me blow, and o'er my soul the waves and billows go. But when the storms beat loudest, and I cry around for help, the Master standeth by, and whispers to my soul, 'Lo, it is I.' Above the tempest wild I hear him say, 'Beyond this darkness lies a perfect day, in every path of thine I lead the way.' So, whether on the hill tops high and fair I dwell, or in the sunless valleys where the shadows lie—what matter? He is there. So where he leads me, I can safely go. And in the blest hereafter I shall know why in his wisdom, he hath led me so.[5]

Faith helps us realize that God has an objective in leaving us on this earth when we feel useless or a burden to others. If we focus on grace from our disease, we can be pleasantly surprised. Even though we cannot be physically cured, we can be spiritually healed. Healing begins when we know God is with us and occasionally it feels as though he is sitting next to us. His presence is so comforting and right that we need not say a word. We can give others the precious gift of our prayers, and if appropriate, fragments of spiritual wisdom that may help them. By giving ourselves over to prayer and accompanying rituals, such as lighting a candle or burning incense, we place the person in the hands of God. During times when pain is so deep that prayer eludes us, holding a cross or a crucifix, or looking at a favorite holy card, can provide spiritual strength and comfort.

Prayer as the Divine Connection

Edith Stein wrote, "Prayer is the communication of the soul with God. God is love, and love is goodness giving itself away. It is a fullness of being that does not want to remain enclosed in itself, but rather to share itself with others, to give itself to them, and to make them happy."[6] Prayer, the essence of our spiritual journey, leads us out of ourselves and into sound action. Edith continues, "Prayer is the highest achievement of which the human spirit is capable. But it is not merely a human achievement. Prayer is a Jacob's ladder in which the human spirit ascends to God and God's grace descends to people."[7]

For some, prayer is the repetition of sounds which have unknown, soothing, or lost significance. For others, praying is rare and limited to dire emergencies. For many, it is the primary way to strengthen a relationship with God and the foundation that supports service to others. Prayer reaches beyond the human scope: past reason, logic, senses, and education. It is a supernatural communication available through faith. "God is our refuge and strength, a very present help in trouble" (Ps. 46:1). When God is our strength, and prayer is our refuge, we recognize how ongoing disease can transport us to a higher level. We entrust God with our disease concerns and find life has a broader horizon because of them.

Prayer can range from singing hymns of praise to being still and receptive to God's word. No matter how busy we are, we pray daily because it is our lifeline to God. In times of prayer, we leave our limited existence and enter something

The Spiritual Dimension

bigger than can ever be imagined. There are no human limits, time, or space, within the majesty of God. What one person knows of him is infinitesimal. In the tenth century, a wise monk described this well. He compared the human knowledge of God to someone standing at the edge of an ocean at midnight trying to see across it with the light from a lantern.

When we are going through difficult treatments, our primary prayer can be, "Dear God, please give me the courage and strength to bear what this day might bring." Conversely, we express thanks when the treatment is over. Prayer shows a beautiful dependence on and gratitude to God. A chronic disease can make us more conscious of God's presence in our lives and consequently, we become better Christians.

To pray for miracles is normal and natural. However, we should be prepared for alternatives. A miracle may not happen or may happen in a way we did not expect. It is good to expect the best, but also to prepare for the worst. Unrealistic expectations distance us from the issues of right now. In practical terms, we can plan for good things but also prepare advance directives and make sure our estate is in order, which means to put who gets what in writing.

If we understand prayer as a sacred refuge, it will be frequently sought and always available. Favorite prayers are a shelter in the silence of sleepless nights when we are plagued by negative disease imagery. We quietly articulate a litany when we are agitated, slowly read an inspirational book when we need support, recite a novena for others who have our disease, or say a chaplet of mercy when we are fearful. Whatever the style, prayer reaches into the depths of our souls and deepens our friendship with God. Often, we pray best when we do not realize we are praying.

Distractions are a common part of authentic prayer. Are these distractions more important than what they are distracting us from? If not we can sweep them away by thinking, not now, maybe later, and getting back to prayer. Hard prayer does not mean God is displeased with us. Severe pain may even make it impossible to pray. God understands. When prayer is difficult, we remain quiet, patient, open, and receptive to grace. Prayer difficulties are common, especially when struggling with the inconsistencies of a chronic disease.

A young man began formation in his lay Carmelite community. He wanted to know the great secrets of mystical prayer. Expecting something very profound, he asked the formation director, who used crutches to walk. He had his pen and paper ready to write her deep spiritual wisdom. The formation director smiled and said the first great secret was—to pray. The young man was brought down to earth. Then the formation director, with a twinkle in her eye, said the second great secret was—to keep at it.

As Healers Who Are Wounded

The depth of love is realized in the crucifixion of Jesus. When we accept God in Christ, we accept him through the cross, our still point in a spinning world, where great evil was overcome by a greater love. In the words of the beloved old hymn of George Bennard, "In that old rugged cross, stained with blood so divine, a wondrous beauty I see. For 'twas on that old cross Jesus suffered and died, to pardon and sanctify me."[8] Through the suffering, death, and resurrection of Jesus, human suffering has great worth and eventually will be over-

The Spiritual Dimension

come. "Suffering, a consequence of original sin, acquires a new meaning; it becomes a participation in the saving work of Jesus."[9]

We hold the cross of Jesus with a firm grip. He keeps us centered on positive aspects of suffering. When we offer our suffering to him, it opens channels of grace that flow into society. United with his suffering our pain integrates into our prayer. The deep distress of disease somehow brings us nearer to God and more empathetic toward those who suffer. A serious disease has a way of helping us distinguish between the things that matter and the things that do not. In union with the holy sacrifice of the Mass, we offer our suffering to Jesus for specific intentions: petitioning God for others such as those in need, the wounded, or the marginalized; and for the conversion of sinners, all of us who consent to do evil. Among serious sins are greed, abuse of people or any other aspect of God's creation, or discrimination against others or groups. We make amends by prayers and actions to atone for sin.

If our disease worsens, our awareness of various aspects of our pain, and the pain of others, can grow. If we are receptive to it, our chronic disease has the ability to transform us into wounded healers. By coping well with its trials and sorrows, we cultivate a greater identification with others who have similar maladies. Words of consolation and encouragement mean more from us because we know, through experience, what others, newly diagnosed, will be going through. It can be very reassuring for a new person on the "no cure" road to share his or her concerns with someone who has been on that road for decades, has had the same concerns, and can help to face them with a positive orientation. In wounded healers authentic hope is alive, and rarely in need of descriptive words, when it is received by others. It is like sunshine on the flowers after a storm. Experiencing a long-term disease, and being able to realistically share aspects of it with others, imparts knowledge with personal depth.

In the Christian tradition there is another dimension within wounded healers called redemptive suffering. This means that wounded healers find a greater purpose in suffering by uniting it with the passion of Jesus and offering it to God in reparation for the evils within humanity. Jesus redeemed all humanity by offering the sufferings of his passion to God the Father. As wounded healers, through offering our sufferings and prayers, we participate in the ongoing work of redemption. We help bring God's love to wherever it is most needed. The love that a wounded healer receives from God through faith is given to others through a listening heart and sincere prayers. Daily prayer sustains a wounded healer's love beyond affective fluctuations that occur in a relationship with God. Prayer is love manifest. Isn't it consoling to hear that someone is praying for us? Wounded healers can pray for those near and far who suffer and have no one to pray for them. A wounded healer's heart can reach out and enfold all hurting people in prayer.

As We Forgive Those Who Hurt Us

When we have a chronic disease, we will meet people in health care who rub us the wrong way. The office nurse who did not return our call. Misinformation about the reason for a visit to a health care professional. The front office person who forgot to put our appointment in the computer. Encounters with aggravating people teach us the importance of not seeking revenge, holding a grudge, or continually repeating an annoying incident in our mind. To release irritants and replace them with forgiveness is an absolute necessity. We cannot move forward without it. To maintain peace of mind, we strive to decrease hurtful or negative mindsets toward people in the past, or present, whom we believe have wronged us. If our hearts are liberated from the refusal to forgive others or ourselves, we identify life lessons more distinctly and see spiritual signs more clearly. As we rise above whatever is holding us down about our chronic disease, we learn that forgiveness and compassion are stronger than anger and indifference. Forgiveness moves us toward personal authenticity, and nearer to God, and others.

Self-forgiveness is needed before we can appropriately forgive others. When forgiving ourselves becomes a daily habit, it lightens the weight of our disease because it releases us from bitterness, hatred, anger, or other self-defeating disease-related defense mechanisms.

Forgiveness is beyond a feeling. It involves daily decisions that take discipline and work, and does not always come naturally or easily. We ask God for help and learn to take steps to prevent an unforgiving state of mind from gaining momentum. In the healthcare industry we find loving as well as unloving people. The more unloving a person is, the more he or she is in need of love. Therefore, we pardon them and place them in the heart of God. Our disease is easier to bear when we banish from our mind dismal thoughts about refusing to forgive ourselves and others.

Courage through Chronic Disease

It was in a church in Munich that I saw him—a balding, heavyset man in a gray overcoat, a brown felt hat clutched between his hands. People were filing out of the basement room where I had just spoken, moving along the rows of wooden chairs to the door at the rear. It was 1947, and I had come from Holland to defeated Germany with the message that God forgives ... And that's where I saw him, working his way forward, against the others. One moment I saw the overcoat and the brown hat; the next, a blue uniform and a visored cap with its skull and crossbones. It came back with a rush: the huge room with its harsh overhead lights; the pathetic pile of dresses and shoes in the center of the floor; the shame of walking naked past this man. I could see my sister's frail form ahead of me, ribs sharp beneath the parchment skin. *Betsie, how thin you were!* The place was Ravensbruck, and the man who was making his way forward had been a guard—one of the most cruel guards. Now he was in front of me, hand thrust out. "A fine message, Fraulein! How good it is to know that, as you say, all our sins are at the bottom of the sea!" And I, who had spoken so glibly of forgiveness, fumbled in my pocketbook rather than take that hand. He would not remember me, of course—how could he remember one prisoner among those thousands of women? But I remembered him, and the leather crop swinging from his belt. I was face to face with one of my captors and my blood seemed to freeze. "You mentioned Ravensbruck in your talk," he was saying. "I was a guard there." No, he did not remember me. "But since that time," he went on, "I have become a Christian. I know that God has forgiven me for the cruel things I did there, but I would like to hear it from your lips as well Fraulein." —again the hand came out,— "will you forgive me?". ... I wrestled with the most difficult thing I had ever had to do ... And still I stood there with the coldness clutching my heart. But forgiveness is not an emotion. I knew that too. Forgiveness is an act of the will, and the will can function regardless of the temperature of the heart. "*Jesus, help me!*" I prayed silently. "*I can lift my hand. You supply the feeling.*" And so woodenly, mechanically, I thrust my hand into the one stretched out to me. And as I did, an incredible thing took place. The current started in my shoulder, raced down my arm, sprang into our joined hands. And then this healing warmth seemed to flood my whole being, bringing tears to my eyes. "I forgive you, brother." I cried. "With all my heart." For a long moment, we grasped each other's hands, the former guard and the former prisoner. I had never known God's love so intensely as I did then.[10]

Corrie's forgiveness story is outstanding. She acknowledged her deep hurt and affirmed her profound pain. She saw the guard beyond the extraordinary painful things he did. Forgiveness is the most profound form of love and love is the linchpin that holds humanity together.

Looking for Jesus Within and Without

Jesus is within us. In her spiritual classic the *Interior Castle*, Teresa of Avila sees the soul of a grace-filled person as a beautiful crystal castle with seven mansions. The seventh mansion is at the center of the soul where Jesus, the King of Glory, resides. The bright light of grace emanates from this room. Outside of the castle everything is foul and dark, symbolic of evil and sin. Teresa sees the spiritual journey as a journey from the deep dark of evil to the bright light of God. She asserts that we never stand still on the spiritual path. We are always moving forward or backward.

There are many ways to find Jesus. A few examples are the following: Pray daily. Ponder a parable or other story from the Bible. If our health permits, fast one day a month. Do a charitable deed once a week. Share a personal spiritual experience with trusted others. Start a collection of prayer cards. Read stories about saintly Christians. If our disease is acting up, think of Mary at the foot of the cross. She, the mother of sorrows, is our mother too. What would it be like to look at Jesus through Mary's eyes?

Ways to find Jesus are innumerable. We choose what is best for our level of well-being, or what fits our present spiritual needs. John of the Cross advises us, "There is much to fathom in Christ, for he is like an abundant mine with many recesses of treasures, so that however deep men go, they never reach the end or bottom, but rather in every recess find new veins with new riches everywhere. On this account St. Paul said of Christ: 'In Christ dwells all treasures and wisdom'" (Col. 2:3).[11]

Laura, an elderly woman, slowly gets out of her car. It has been her habit to attend daily early Mass and she has done so for many years. However, the years are catching up as she feels more limitations from her chronic disease. It takes her longer to get ready for Mass. She tires easily. Consequently, she moves slowly to the church door. The pain and unsteady gait causes her to be more attentive to her walking. Walking was a breeze in previous years, but now she has to think about it and avoids chatting while walking. She does not want to fall and uses a walker to steady herself. Pain is like an old familiar friend these days, yet she has to admit that sometimes she gets perturbed with her friend. Well, maybe it is more than sometimes. She enters the church and goes to her usual place. She sits through Mass. At communion, she shuffles carefully up the aisle. After the Mass, she remains still, resting her head on her hands absorbed in quiet prayer. The priest gazes at the woman in the stillness after Mass. He ponders how she was active in so many ministries in the past but is now engaged in her most vital ministry. He muses that the woman's love of prayer brings strength and peace to this church. She is important to the parish, more important than she realizes. This woman and others like her, although not involved in busy parish activities, are the backbone of the parish because of their fidelity to unwavering prayer.

Finding the Blessings Everywhere

Blessings come in all shapes and sizes and can originate in times from great joy to great suffering. Helen Steiner Rice was known as America's beloved inspirational poet laureate. She penned this poem:

> Blessings come in many guises
> that God alone in love devises.
> And sickness which we dread so much
> can bring a very healing touch.
> For often on the wings of pain
> the peace we sought before in vain
> Will come to us with sweet surprise
> for God is merciful and wise.

Courage through Chronic Disease

> And through long hours of tribulation
> God gives us time for meditation.
> And no sickness can be counted loss
> that teaches us to bear our cross.[12]

To bless, in the sense that we bless, means to say positive things that encourage and uplift. Whether a blessing is given in words or in gestures, solemnly or simply, it is a channel of God's grace. The Irish are unsurpassed regarding the bestowal of blessings. A common sense blessing, especially regarding questionable treatment for chronic disease, is: "May you have the hindsight to know where you've been, the foresight to know where you are going, and the insight to know when you have gone too far." Blessings comfort and console during the dark days of our disease. Blessings invoke God to enrich, empower, and protect us, and lessen anxiety and fear about our disease trepidations. God is the source of blessings and the one from whom all blessings flow. We are the messengers of that source. A blessing helps love grow in our hearts especially when we feel unlovable because of our chronic physical difficulties. The more we count the blessings in our day, the less we dwell on our physical limitations.

Physical problems can cause us to slow down. However, slowness can be a blessing in disguise. It is better to do things slowly and well, then quickly and chaotically. An unhurried pace allows us to see beautiful things we never noticed in the fast lane, such as a flower in a crannied rock, or a rainbow in the sky. A quiet gaze at natural wonders can guide us toward God, and in his light we ponder where we stand, what is right, and the course to take. We live in a speedy society; however, slow is often good and, in many ways, yet to be valued.

The Spiritual Dimension

An unexpected blessing is when others see good qualities in us that we do not see, such as genuineness, diligence, or fortitude. When they bring it to our attention, we are delightfully surprised since we never expected this compliment. Blessings are small sunbeams of grace, that reassure us of God's love for us and sustain our understanding of our value as human beings.

In 2 Corinthians 12:10, Paul the apostle said, "For when I am weak, then I am strong." To be strong indicates the ability to do things by ourselves, without help from anyone. We lift heavy objects, have unending energy, and are in control. In our weakness we can't make things happen on our own. Therefore, we surrender to God, let him lead the way, and rely on his strength. We depend on him, the almighty Father, as Jesus did in his passion and death on the cross. In the most vulnerable of weaknesses, he unveiled the greatest act of love that helps us to trust him and to bear our physical limitations gracefully. With love we cannot possibly comprehend, Jesus carries our pain with us. Weakness brings us to prayer, and, as weak Christians, we grow in compassion, serve with kind action, and let our actions bring us back to prayer.

A lifelong disease journey can unfurl innovative blessings. We meet new friends, discover new interests, or find new hobbies. There is strength in our broken places. We move beyond instant excuses that hold us back (I cannot do that) to reasons that push us ahead (I'll try that). Small problem frustrations diminish in the light of big problems that were overcome. Because we have dealt with serious difficulties, we have a greater capacity for managing or working with people who have different views by finding a common ground rather than arguing about who is right. Thus we go from the conflictive individual "I" to the uniting communal "we."

A beautiful blessing on the spiritual journey is a change in the way we think about people who have physical problems. First, we focus on the positive aspects and goodness of their personhood, and down the list, we acknowledge their physical concern. The young man with an exuberance for living outshines his significant limp. A middle-aged woman with an easy smile and upbeat persona surpasses her chronic cough. The infusion nurse who offers encouraging words before she starts an IV goes beyond her cancer.

Responses to how God is present in the midst of suffering could be philosophical, poetical or theological. However, a simple Christian response is that in suffering, God gives us a readily available hope. The crucifix exemplifies that Christian love always rekindles hope and resurgent hope gives life. No matter how hard it is to live through suffering, we cannot rule out the possibility that stronger life is in its midst. We grow in the mystery of suffering and it brings us closer to God. In Romans 5:3–5, Paul describes suffering as a continuum of blessings: "More than that, we rejoice in our sufferings, knowing that suffering produces endurance, and endurance produces character, and character produces hope, and hope does not disappoint us because God's love has been poured into our hearts through the Holy Spirit which has been given to us."

With our chronic disease we bask in, and strive to live out, the love and mercy of God. This helps us to see everything as a blessing. Karl Rahner, a renowned theologian, said shortly before his death at the age of eighty: "The real high

The Spiritual Dimension

point of my life is still to come. I mean the abyss of the mystery of God into which one lets oneself fall in complete confidence of being caught up by God's love and mercy forever." [13]

Our greatest blessing is Jesus, who is far beyond anyone we have known or can imagine. No one loves us more than Jesus. No one heals us more deeply than Jesus. No peace can be more deeply felt than the peace of Christ. No one sees the depths and the fruits of our pain more profoundly than Jesus. We do not become overwhelmed when we are afflicted, perplexed, or bewildered by our physical limitations because Jesus is truly with us. And because of him, we do not lose hope and keep moving forward to God and with God.

The mystical doctor, John of the Cross, observed that he saw a river over which every soul must pass to reach the kingdom of heaven, and the name of that river was suffering. And he saw the boat which carried souls across the river, and the name of that boat was love. As we navigate this river, may we remain steadfast in Christ, and be signs of his love, until we reach the shores of heaven.

> Lord, make me an instrument of your peace;
> where there is hatred, let me sow love;
> where there is injury, pardon;
> where there is doubt, faith;
> where there is despair, hope;
> where there is darkness, light;
> and where there is sadness, joy.
> Grant that I may not so much
> seek to be consoled as to console;
> to be understood as to understand,

to be loved as to love;
for it is in giving that we receive,
it is in pardoning that we are pardoned,
and it is in dying
that we are born to eternal life.

Francis of Assisi

Notes

1. Anthea Dove, *Touched by God* (Dublin, Ireland: The Columba Press, 2012), 35.
2. Homily of his Holiness Pope Benedict XVI, St. Peter's Square, Sunday, April 24, 2005.
3. John Paul II, *Salvifici doloris*, February 11, 1984, n. 27.
4. Thomas Merton, *Thoughts in Solitude* (New York, NY: Farrar Straus and Giroux-Macmillan, 1956), 79.
5. John F. Chaplain, *He Leadeth Me*, (leaflet) (Addison IL: Bible Truth Publishers, n.d.) https://bibletruthpublishers.com/he-leadeth-me-poetry-leaflets-11-point-type/john-f-chaplain/pd7962.
6. Edith Stein, *The Hidden Life: Hagiographic Essays, Meditations, Spiritual Texts*, trans. Waltraut Stein, Lucy Gelber, and Michael Linssen: *The Collected Works of Edith Stein*, vol. 4 (Washington, D.C.: ICS Publications, 1992), 38.
7. Stein, *The Hidden Life*, 38.
8. George Bennard, 1913, "The Old Rugged Cross," Timeless Truths Free Online Library, https://library.timelesstruths.org/music/The_Old_Rugged_Cross/.
9. *Catechism of the Catholic Church*, 1521.
10. Corrie ten Boom with Jamie Buckingham, *Tramp for the Lord* (Fort Washington, PA: CLC Publications, 1974), 55–57. The ten Boom family harbored Jews in their Holland home during the Nazi persecution, helping nearly eight hundred people reach safety. A secret room became the hiding place for the Jews until the family was discovered and arrested by the Gestapo in 1944. *The Hiding Place* is a book and movie that describes Corrie's story.

11. St. John of the Cross, "The Spiritual Canticle," in *The Collected Works of St. John of the Cross*, trans. Kieran Kavanaugh, OCD, and Otilio Rodriguez, OCD (Washington DC: ICS Publications, 1973), 551, stanza 37 l. 4.

12. Helen Steiner Rice, "There Are Blessings in Everything," in *The Poems and Prayers of Helen Steiner Rice*, (Fleming H. Revell, a division of Baker Book House Company, 2003): 134.

13. Karl Rahner, *Faith in a Wintery Season: Conversations and Interviews with Karl Rahner in the Last Years of His Life* (New York, NY: Crossroad, 1990), 38.

Printed in the USA
CPSIA information can be obtained
at www.ICGtesting.com
LVHW080948041123
762823LV00006B/15